Ch 1,2,9
169-184

RECENT ADVANCES
IN NEUROLOGY AND
NEUROPSYCHIATRY

RECENT ADVANCES IN NEUROLOGY AND NEUROPSYCHIATRY

EIGHTH EDITION

Edited by

The late LORD BRAIN

D.M., F.R.C.P., F.R.S.

Formerly Consulting Neurologist to the London Hospital:
Consulting Physician to the Maida Vale Hospital for
Nervous Diseases, London

and

MARCIA WILKINSON

D.M., F.R.C.P.

Consultant Neurologist, Elizabeth Garrett Anderson
Hospital and the Hackney Group of Hospitals. Director,
Regional Neurological Unit, Eastern Hospital, Hackney
London

With 42 Illustrations

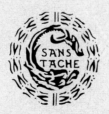

WILLIAMS AND WILKINS COMPANY
BALTIMORE

First Edition	.	.	.	.	1929
Second Edition	.	.	.	.	1930
Third Edition	.	.	.	.	1934
Fourth Edition	.	.	.	.	1940
Fifth Edition	.	.	.	.	1945
Reprinted	.	.	.	.	1946
Reprinted	.	.	.	.	1947
Translated into Italian					
Translated into Roumanian					
Sixth Edition	.	.	.	.	1955
Seventh Edition		.	.	.	1962
Eighth Edition	.	.	.	.	1969

ISBN 0 7000 1393 8

Printed in Great Britain at the Pitman Press, Bath

PREFACE

LORD BRAIN was working on this edition of the book at the time of his death in December 1966. It was his wish and that of the other contributors that this edition should be published as he had planned it. I have endeavoured to carry this out in collaboration with Dr. Michael Brain, who as his father's literary executor has assisted me in the production of this edition.

The book has been extensively rewritten and contains much new material. Lord Brain's own contributions, some of his last writings, are a chapter on Disorders of Memory, a subject in which he was particularly interested, Otoneurology, Disorders of Cerebral Circulation, and a chapter on the Carcinomatous Neuromyopathies written in conjunction with Dr. P. B. Croft and Dr. Marcia Wilkinson. The chapter on the Cerebral Circulation was incomplete at the time of his death but was considered of sufficient interest to be included without major alteration. I am most grateful to Miss P. K. L. Orton for her assistance with the chapter on Otoneurology.

New contributions to this edition include a chapter on Disorders of Muscle by Professor John N. Walton, The Surgery of Cerebral Hæmorrhage by Mr. R. T. Johnson and one on Stereotaxic Surgery by Mr. John Hankinson. Dr. M. V. Driver has again contributed a chapter on Electroencephalography and Dr. David Sutton one on Neuroradiology.

I should like to express my appreciation to the publishers for their unfailing courtesy and help in the production of this edition.

MARCIA WILKINSON

CONTRIBUTORS

The late LORD BRAIN, DM., FRCP., FRS. Former Consulting Neurologist to The London Hospital and Consulting Physician to the Maida Vale Hospital for Nervous Diseases, London.

M. C. BRAIN, DM., FRCP. Lecturer in Hæmatology and Medicine, Royal Postgraduate Medical School, London.

P. B. CROFT, BSC., BM., BCH., MRCP. Consultant Neurologist to the Tottenham Group of Hospitals, the Whittington Hospital, London, the Lister Hospital, Hitchin, and the Queen Elizabeth II Hospital, Welwyn Garden City.

M. V. DRIVER, MB., BS., PH.D. Consultant Neurophysiologist, the Bethlem Royal and Maudsley Hospitals, London.

JOHN HANKINSON, MB., BS., FRCS. Lecturer in Neurological Surgery, The University of Newcastle upon Tyne. Consultant Neurological Surgeon, The Royal Victoria Infirmary and the Regional Neurological Centre, Newcastle upon Tyne.

R. T. JOHNSON, OBE., FRCS. Director, University Department of Neurosurgery, Royal Infirmary, Manchester.

DAVID SUTTON, MD., FRCP., FFR., DMRD. Director, Radiological Department, St. Mary's Hospital, London, W.2. Consultant Radiologist, Maida Vale Hospital (the National Hospitals for Nervous Diseases). Teacher in Radiology, University of London.

JOHN N. WALTON, TD., MD., FRCP. Professor of Neurology, University of Newcastle upon Tyne. Neurologist, Regional Neurological Centre, Newcastle General Hospital. Physician in Neurology, Royal Victoria Infirmary, Newcastle upon Tyne.

MARCIA WILKINSON, DM., FRCP. Consultant Neurologist, Elizabeth Garrett Anderson Hospital and the Hackney Group of Hospitals. Director, Regional Neurological Unit, Eastern Hospital, Hackney, E.9.

CONTENTS

CHAPTER 1

DISORDERS OF MEMORY

The late LORD BRAIN

DURING recent years, many clinical and pathological observations have been made which throw light upon the situation of cerebral lesions likely to interfere with memory. The first of these is the hippocampal gyrus (Fig. 1). Scoville and Milner (1957) have observed in ten cases of bilateral hippocampal excision, an amnesia unrelated to any deterioration of the intellect or personality of the subjects. Milner (1958) observed an equally severe memory loss in two patients who underwent excision of the left hippocampal region only, and assumed that in these cases the same area on the opposite side must previously have been damaged, as the result of which the subsequent unilateral excision had the same effect as a bilateral excision. Walker (1957) reports four cases of recent memory impairment after unilateral temporal lobe lesions, and asks why severe memory loss should occur in only 10 to 15 per cent of temporal lobe operations on either the dominant or the non-dominant side. He suggests that these

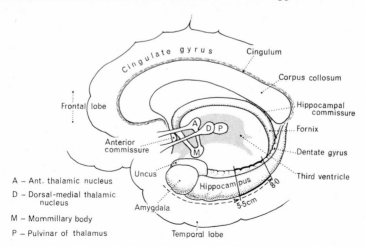

A – Ant. thalamic nucleus
D – Dorsal-medial thalamic nucleus
M – Mammillary body
P – Pulvinar of thalamus

Figure 1.

differences may depend upon individual variations in the use of imagery, and that a severe memory loss may occur in those using predominantly visual imagery.

Bickford *et al.* (1958) report three cases of patients in whom changes in memory function resulted from stimulation below the cortical surface of the temporal lobe. In one patient stimulation in the region of the superior temporal gyrus evoked a past experience. In two other patients, stimulation in the general region of the posterior part of the middle temporal gyrus below the surface produced a syndrome of loss of memory for recent events up to several days, with normal recall for events preceding the amnesia. The severity of the amnesia depended on the duration of the stimulation and complete recovery occurred in from one minute to two hours.

The evidence based upon surgical resection of the whole or part of one or both temporal lobes indicates that gross impairment of recent memory results usually from bilateral lesions of the hippo-campus, particularly the area between 5 and 8 cm from the tip of the temporal lobe. Unilateral lesions do not usually have this effect though they sometimes do. Bilateral removal of the uncus and amygdala does not impair memory.

Penfield (Penfield and Jasper, 1954, Penfield, 1958) has reported many instances of the vocation of memories of past events by the electrical stimulation of the temporal cortex in patients operated on for temporal lobe epilepsy under local anæsthesia.

Another structure which has been implicated is the fornix (Fig. 1). Sweet, Talland and Ervin (1959) have reported cases of amnesia which they attributed to lesions of the fornix, but the evidence for its importance in relation to memory, recently reviewed by Ojemann (1964) appears inconclusive. It has been divided on both sides and also been congenitally absent without any impairment of memory.

Impairment of memory is an important element in Korsakoff's syndrome, to be discussed more fully below, hence the relevance of the site of the lesions in Korsakoff's syndrome. Adams, Collins and Victor (1962) and Victor (1965) state that the only constant lesions are in the medial parts of the medial dorsal, pulvinar and antero-ventral nuclei of the thalamus, the mammillary bodies, and the terminal portions of the fornices. Barbizet (1963) regards the mammillary bodies as particularly important in relation to memory defects (Fig. 1).

Some light is thrown on this problem by more diffuse lesions. Thus, Williams and Pennybacker (1954) investigated 180 patients with intracranial tumour and found that memory impairment was most common and specific when the lesion involved the floor or the walls of the third ventricle, and Delay, Brion and Derouesné (1964) report three cases of intracranial tumour with impairment of memory and review the literature, coming to the conclusion that memory disturbances occur when the tumour interrupts a circuit running from the hippocampus to the mammillary bodies and then to the thalamus, and finally to the cingulate gyrus bilaterally.

Victor, Angevine, Mancall and Fisher (1961) report a case of great interest from the anatomical point of view. Their patient, who was the subject of prolonged study, had a severe loss of recent memory. The cerebral lesions to which this was attributed were bilateral infarctions of the infero-medial portions of the temporal lobes and related structures, particularly the hippocampal formation, fornix and mamillary bodies. The uncus, amygdaloid body and terminal digitations of the hippocampus were unaffected on either side.

Encephalitis sometimes leads to severe impairment of recent memory. Rose and Symonds (1960) have reported four patients who, after what was presumed to be an attack of encephalitis, were left with a retrograde amnesia for several years before the onset of the illness, and a severe defect of recent memory with relatively little impairment of other intellectual functions. Reviewing the literature they conclude that in their patients the lesion must have had a selective incidence upon the hippocampus, fornix, or mammillary bodies. Brierley, Corsellis, Hierons and Nevin (1960) have reported three fatal cases of subacute encephalitis of later adult life, in two of which loss of memory was mentioned in the history. The general picture was one of a progressive dementia ending in one or several brief periods of coma. The pathological changes were those of a severe encephalitis concentrated in the limbic areas of the brain, which was taken to include the uncus and the amygdaloid nucleus, the hippocampus and dentate gyrus, the limen insulæ and hippocampal and cingulate gyri.

Finally, Whitty and Lewin (1960) have described loss of recent memory in the confusional state following cingulectomy. The localization of the lesions responsible for impairment of recent memory has been reviewed by Ojemann (1964).

In summary, then, surgical excision of an area of both hippocampal gyri extending between 5 and 8 cm from the tip of the temporal lobe appears invariably to cause permanent loss of recent memory, and unilateral excision of the same area sometimes does so. Loss of recent memory has also followed more diffuse lesions sparing the hippocampal gyri but involving the fornices, the mammillary bodies and parts of the thalamus. It has also resulted from surgical lesions of the cingulate gyri. There is considerable evidence that all these structures play a part in the same process which utilizes a complex pathway extending from the hippocampal gyri, probably through the fornices to the mammillary bodies, thence to the thalamus and finally to the cingulate gyri, though how these structures are functionally related is unknown.

THE TRAUMATIC AMNESIAS

Two forms of amnesia may follow a head injury: these are retrograde amnesia, RA, i.e. amnesia for events which occurred before the injury, and post-traumatic amnesia, PTA, which is the loss of memory for events occurring after the injury. Russell (1959) has published a study of memory and learning in which he discusses both retrograde and post-traumatic amnesia. Brief retrograde amnesia is very common after concussion, and in his view indicates a block between sensory reception and the process of retention for future recall. A long period of retrograde amnesia is usually associated with a long post-traumatic amnesia and indicates severe damage which affects recent more than distant memory. More recently, Russell and Smith (1961) have analyzed the data relating to PTA in a series of 1,766 cases of closed head injury. They divided their patients into four groups. Group A was an acute group with admission to hospital within three days of the injury. Group B was a subacute group with admission within three weeks of the injury. Group C was a chronic group with admission more than three weeks after the injury, and Group D a similar chronic group, differing from C only in that the patients had been selected for admission on account of substantial injuries and symptoms. Russell and Smith classify the period of PTA as follows: nil, less than one hour, 1–24 hours, 1–7 days, and more than 7 days. They found six signs or symptoms, the incidence of which consistently increased with longer PTAs in all four groups. These positively correlated features were: fracture of the skull, motor disorder, anosmia, dysphasia, memory and/or calculation defect, and a retrograde amnesia lasting more than 30 minutes. On the other hand, there were three clinical features which showed a consistently random relationship to the duration of the PTA, namely, anxiety and depression, giddiness without vertigo, and headache. Russell and Smith found both in their series and in a series of 1,000 cases, the details of which were provided by Lewin, that the incidence of long PTA systematically increased with age in each of the four populations, and, further, that the interaction of age and the duration of the PTA provided a more reliable assessment of the severity of closed head injury than when one of the two factors was taken into consideration alone. It was thought that the signs which correlated positively with the duration of the PTA in all four groups were those of a brain lesion, whereas those which did not were not.

Russell (1959) points out that there must be some neurological difference between a brief RA and one lasting for several days, as may happen in some cases of severe head injury with a long PTA. The long RA differs from the memory disorders of organic dementia in that in the latter not only are recent memories lost, but also the ability to recall events from day to day, whereas in most cases of head injury this faculty returns to normal after recovery from the confusion.

What is the explanation of retrograde amnesia? Russell (1959) writes as follows: "The almost constant occurrence of RA after concussion indicates that the injury, though it cannot have time to prevent what is last seen or heard from reaching the sensorium, does completely prevent its retention for future recall. The latter process presumably requires a few seconds of time for completion. The occasional occurrence of a vision of events within the RA indicates that in these cases some form of registration has occurred with great vividness which, though it can never be properly retained for later recall, can reproduce itself from a relatively low level in the form of a momentary "vision." The injury in such a case appears to have blocked the process of retention half-way. The variations in the RA during recovery of full consciousness seem to be specially significant. Distant memories return first, and loss of memory for the previous few years may, for a time, be so complete, that the patient believes himself to be several years younger. After severe injury there may be a permanent RA of several days duration, which may include events of great importance to the patient . . . We are therefore forced to the conclusion that as memories become older they become more strongly established, irrespective of their importance to the individual, while recent memories are relatively liable to traumatic extinction, however important they may be . . . It seems likely that memory of events is not a static process. If it were, then distant memories would surely fade gradually and be the more vulnerable to the effects of injury. On the contrary, when the brain is injured, these distant memories are the least vulnerable. It seems that the mere existence of the brain as a functioning organ must strengthen the roots of distant memories. The normal activity of the brain must steadily strengthen distant memories so that with the passage of time, these become less vulnerable to the effects of head injury." Russell thus concludes that memory depends on an active neuronal mechanism which never rests.

Gooddy (1964) has proposed an interesting hypothesis to explain retrograde amnesia. He likens the process of memory to the operation of a tape-recorder, upon which current events make a permanent impression, which is then stored. He suggests that if the area of tape of a tape-recorder which is at the moment recording, is exposed to an unusually violent electrical disturbance, this must spread along the tape into the region on which the most recent record has been made and obliterate this. Something of this kind, he suggests, happens when a head injury obliterates the most recently recorded memories and so causes retrograde amnesia.

AMNESIA FOR CURRENT EVENTS

The term "amnesia for current events," also known as loss of recent memory and loss of ongoing memory, describes a condition in which the patient, who is otherwise mentally normal, is unable to recall what has just happened to him. Milner (1958) reporting two such patients, said that they "show a very gross impairment of memory for all events subsequent to operation, and they are unable to recall test material after a lapse of five minutes or less, if their attention has been diverted to another topic in the meantime. The retention difficulty is not specific to any one kind of material, but is quite general, affecting stories, drawings and numbers, and cutting across any distinction between verbal and perceptual material or between one sense modality and another." Victor *et al.* (1961) say of their patient that his "ability to recall recent events and to learn and retain new facts were both seriously affected. He would ask the same question over and over again. He spent hours watching baseball on television, but as soon as the set was turned off, he was unable to remember the score or any other detail of the game. However, he was able to recall correctly the highlights of games which had been played many years before. He could not remember whether he had smoked a cigarette or simply put it away . . . During this period he was still able to play bridge adequately and actually taught his nephew the game of solitaire, but he was unable to learn new card games, such as canasta." There are, however, slight exceptions to the amnesia. Both the patient of Victor *et al.* and one of my own were able to recall events with a strong emotional tone which had occurred after the onset of their amnesia.

There is ample evidence that in its pure form, amnesia for current events is not associated with any other psychological disability. Remote memories are well preserved, though there may be some persistent retrograde amnesia for the events which preceded the illness or operation giving rise to the persistent memory defects. Attention, concentration, and reasoning ability are normal, but the patient fails seriously on the Wechsler Memory Scale. The retention of memory for remote events includes that for skills acquired before the illness, hence Milner's two patients were both able to earn their living, one as a glove-cutter and the other as a draughtsman.

As stated above, the lesion responsible for amnesia for current events is situated somewhere along the pathway from the hippocampal gyrus through the fornix to the mammillary bodies, optic thalamus and cingulate gyrus. When the amnesia occurs without other symptoms, it is probably most frequently in the hippocampal gyri. In its pure form, it may result from surgical excision of part of both hippocampal gyri, ischæmic lesions due to cerebral atheroma within the terminal area of supply of the vertebro-basilar system, or rarely, acute encephalitis. More diffuse lesions are likely to produce Korsakoff's syndrome, which will now be considered.

KORSAKOFF'S SYNDROME

Korsakoff's syndrome is characterized predominantly by an amnesia for current events and confabulation, with which various symptoms of a confusional state may be associated. There is also a retrograde amnesia of variable length for events preceding the illness.

Pathology and Ætiology

Korsakoff's syndrome was first recognized in association with chronic alcoholism and it is now known that in such cases the causal factor is a deficiency of vitamin B1 (aneurin, thiamin). Deficiency of this vitamin also produces Wernicke's encephalopathy. In the opinion of Victor (1965) the two are identical, and he therefore speaks of the Korsakoff-Wernicke syndrome. According to Victor, the topography of the lesions is remarkably constant, the principal changes being located in the medial parts of the medial, dorsal, pulvinar and antero-ventral thalamic nuclei, the mammillary bodies and the terminal portions of the fornices. Minor and inconstant changes are also found in other thalamic nuclei and the hypothalamus, the brain stem, and the anterior lobe of the cerebellum. The lesions consist of loss of medullated fibres and nerve cells, large numbers of adventitial histiocytes and microglia, increased cellularity of capillaries and small blood vessels, and an increased number of fibrous astrocytes. Evidence of hæmorrhage was noted in approximately 20 per cent of cases but was seldom conspicuous.

It would appear from what has been said above that the pathological changes responsible for the symptoms in Korsakoff's syndrome are those in the fornices, the mammillary bodies and the thalamic nuclei. It follows that other pathological changes involving the same structures are likely to produce a similar clinical picture. Korsakoff's syndrome therefore may result from head injury, anoxia, carbon monoxide poisoning, epilepsy, electro-convulsive therapy, acute encephalitis, dementia paralytica and other forms of dementia, intracranial tumour, cerebral arteriosclerosis, and the operation of cingulectomy.

Symptoms

The symptoms of Korsakoff's syndrome have long been familiar and the subject has recently been reviewed by Lewis (1961). The amnesia for current events is similar to that described above; the patient has no recollection of what has recently happened to him. In confabulating, the patient describes experiences which either have not happened or have not happened when he says they did. Whitty and Lewin (1960), studying the post-cingulectomy confusional state, suggest that the confabulation may not be pure invention but may be the result of misplacing memories in time, and Russell (1959) has put forward a similar explanation of confabulation in post-traumatic amnesic syndromes. Lewis draws attention to the dream-like quality of confabulation in some cases of Korsakoff's syndrome and also the importance of emotional factors in distorting or repressing memories. There is a retrograde amnesia, which may extend to years, for events preceding the onset of the illness. Temporal order and temporal relationships are invariably disturbed, and disorders of perception and attention are present. These have been studied by Talland (1958, 1959, 1960a and b), Talland and Ekdahl (1959) and Talland (1965). The treatment of Korsakoff's syndrome is that of the causal disorder.

TRANSIENT GLOBAL AMNESIA

Fisher and Adams (1964) have recently drawn attention to a syndrome characterized by sudden temporary amnesia, usually of a few hours duration, followed by complete restoration to the previous state of health. Fisher and Adams report 17 cases and I have myself seen 9. In Fisher and Adams' series, 13 of the patients were men and 4 were women, all were middle-aged or elderly. Among causal factors mentioned by Fisher and Adams the attack developed in two women after bathing in the sea and two men had taken showerbaths. The attack followed bathing in three of my patients, in one of whom two attacks occurred, both after bathing. Two of Fisher and Adams' patients and one of mine had an attack after sexual intercourse. No other significant precipitating factors appeared. In 4 of their cases the patient was aware that something was wrong, in the remaining 13 he was unaware of this, but it was noticed by his family or friends.

Conversation with the patient during an attack showed that there was an amnesia, often patchy, for the events of the previous days, weeks, months, or even years. Recovery usually occurred gradually over a period of one to several hours, during which time the period of retrograde amnesia progressively shrank. After recovery the patient was left with complete amnesia for the period of the attack and there was also a period of retrograde amnesia for events preceding the attack.

No patient in Fisher and Adams' series or in my own showed any evidence of an epileptic attack at the onset, nor was there any weakness, paralysis, or sensory disturbance relating to the limbs, nor aphasia. Behaviour during the attack was always quiet and there was no restlessness or automatic activity. On clinical examination there was no evidence of any organic neurological disorder related to the attack. Such routine laboratory investigations as were carried out were normal. In Fisher and Adams' series, an electroencephalogram was obtained after the end of the amnesia in 13 cases. It was normal in 8 and in the remaining 5 a variety of diffuse or focal abnormalities were observed. Fisher and Adams' follow-up of their patients showed the benign character of the syndrome. The average period of follow-up was approximately three years and only one patient developed a neurological disorder, namely, a moderately severe stroke, seven months after the amnesic episode. My own experience has been similar.

Fisher and Adams discuss the pathogenesis of this syndrome without arriving at any definite conclusion. They begin by noting that "the episodes, by virtue of their brevity, transiency, reversibility, and associated suspension of memory recording, bear a close resemblance to the amnesic spells described in temporal lobe seizures." However, "if epilepsy is the basis, the literature on the subject does not record similar examples," and one might add the complete freedom from a recurrence over a period of years in many cases is strongly against epilepsy. There is a little more evidence that these episodes may be due to transient cerebral ischæmic attacks in view of the age of the patients and the association in some cases with evidence of atheroma. However, the benign outlook is unlike that of cerebral atheroma. Moreover, Fisher reviewed 200 cases of cerebral thrombosis without discovering any instance of attacks of amnesia of this kind. Fisher and Adams conclude that there is no decisive evidence in favour of the view that the amnesic episodes are caused by transient focal cerebral ischæmia or a small stroke. Hysterical amnesia obviously enters into the diagnosis but there are points against this also. Apart from the fact that, as Fisher and Adams point out, psychogenic amnesia has its own distinctive features which are not present in the patients under consideration, hysterical symptoms do not commonly appear for the first time in patients aged between 50 and 70 of previously stable personality. In fact, we need more data before we can elucidate the pathogenesis of this unusual amnesic syndrome.

THE NEUROLOGY OF MEMORY

From all that has been said, it will be clear that the temporal lobe plays an important part in the cerebral organization of memory. Part of the hippocampal gyrus appears to be the start of a pathway through which current experiences are converted into memories. This pathway appears to run from the hippocampal gyri through the fornices to the mammillary bodies and thence to the thalami and cingulate gyri (Fig. 1). It is not suggested that these parts of the brain are concerned with the storage of memories as such: they are rather the route by which experiences are processed or conducted to the areas in which they are ultimately stored. This is consistent with the view, for which there is other evidence, that cortical associational pathways converge on the temporal lobes and that experiences are linked with their emotional components there. Destruction of the hippocampal gyri therefore leads to loss of the capacity to convert current experiences into memories. As a result, the patient becomes unable to remember what has just happened to him.

That the temporal lobe also plays some part in the evocation of memories is suggested by Penfield's observations that electrical stimulation of the temporal cortex in the conscious patient was capable of evoking memories.

How and where memories are stored is little understood. Neurophysiologists, thinking in terms of electrical impulses and synaptic changes, have suggested that memories depend upon reverberating neural circuits. This, however, seems improbable in view of the fact that memories can be retained after electroconvulsive shocks, hypothermia, and narcotics, all of which abolish electrical activity in the nervous system. Recent work illustrating the importance of molecular changes for the storage of genetic information has suggested that similar molecular changes may underlie the storage of memory, but if this is so, it has yet to be shown how such changes are produced by neural impulses, for the storage of memories, and how in turn they are re-converted into neural impulses in the process of recall. There is much evidence that whatever the precise method by which memories are stored, their storage is diffuse in the cerebral hemispheres rather than localized. Lashley (1950, 1960), one of the earliest workers in this field, concludes that the associative connections for memory traces do not extend across the cortex as well-defined arcs or paths. Such arcs are either diffuse through all parts of the cortex, passed by relays through lower centres, or do not exist. Memory disturbances of simple sensory habits follow only upon very extensive experimental destruction, including almost the entire associative cortex. Small lesions, embracing no more than a single associative area do not produce loss of any habit: large lesions produce deterioration which affects a variety of habits, irrespective of the sensory motor elements involved. There is no evidence, therefore, of any restricted localization of specific memory changes in the cortex.

References

ADAMS, R. B., COLLINS, G. H., and VICTOR, M. (1962). *Physiologie de l'Hippocampe*, p. 273. Paris, Editions du Centre National de la Recherche Scientifique.

BARBIZET, J., (1963). *J. Neurol. Neurosurg. Psychiat.* **26**, 127.

BICKFORD, R. C., MULDER, D. W., DODGE, H. W. Jr., SVIEN, H. J., and ROME, H. P. (1958). *Ass. Res. nerv. Dis. Proc.* **36**, 227.

BRIERLEY, J. B., CORSELLIS, J. A. N., HIERONS, R., and NEVIN, S. (1960). *Brain*, **83**, 357.

DELAY, J., BRION, S., DEROUESNÉ, C. (1964). *Rev. neurol.*, **111**, 97.

FISHER, C. M., and ADAMS, R. D. (1964). *Acta neurol. scand.*, **40**, Suppl. 9, pp. 1–83.

GOODDY, W. (1964). *Brain*, **87**, 75.

LASHLEY, K. S. (1950). *Symp. Soc. exp. Biol.*, **4**, 454.

LASHLEY, K. S. (1960). In *The Neuropsychology of Lashley*, Ed. F. A. Beach, D. O. Hebb, C. T. Morgan, and H. W. Nissen, p. 482, *et seq.*, New York, McGraw-Hill.

LEWIS, A. (1961). *Proc. roy. Soc. Med.*, 54, 955.

MILNER, B. (1958). *Ass. Res. nerv. Dis. Proc.*, **36**, 244.

OJEMANN, R. G. (1964). *Neuro-Sciences Research Programme Bulletin*, **2**, 77.

PENFIELD, W., and JASPER, H. (1954). *Epilepsy and the Functional Anatomy of the Human Brain*, p. 125. London, Churchill.

PENFIELD, W. (1958). In *Neurological Basis of Behaviour*, ed. G. E. W. Wolstenholme and C. M. O'Connor, p. 149. London, Churchill.

ROSE, F. C., and SYMONDS, C. P. (1960), *Brain*, **83**, 195.

RUSSELL, W. R. (1959). *Brain Memory Learning*, Oxford.

RUSSELL, W. R., and SMITH, A. (1961). *Arch. Neurol (Chic.)*, **5**, 4.

SCOVILLE, W. B., and MILNER, B. (1957). *J. Neurol. Neurosurg. Psychiat.*, **20**, 11.

SWEET, W. H., TALLAND, G. A., and ERVIN, F. R. (1959). *Trans. Amer. neurol. Ass.*, **76**.

TALLAND, G. A. (1958). *J. nerv. ment. Dis.*, **127**, 197.

TALLAND, G. A. (1959). *J. abnorm. soc. Psychol.*, **59**, 10.

TALLAND, G. A. (1960a). *J. nerv. ment. Dis.*, **130**, 16.

TALLAND, G. A. (1960b). *J. nerv. ment. Dis.*, **130**, 366.

TALLAND, G. A. (1965). *Deranged Memory*. New York, Academic Press.

TALLAND, G. A., and EKDAHL, M. (1959). *J. nerv. ment. Dis.*, **129**, 391.

VICTOR, M. (1965). In "The Remote Effects of Cancer on the Nervous System." Ed. Lord Brain and F. H. Norris, p. 134. New York, Grune and Stratton.

VICTOR, M., ANGEVINE, J. B. Jr., MANCALL, E. L., and FISHER, C. M. (1961). *Arch. Neurol. (Chic.)*, **5**, 244.

WALKER, A. E. (1957). *Arch. Neurol. Psychiat. (Chic.)*, **78**, 543.

WHITTY, C. W. M., and LEWIN, W. (1960). *Brain*, **83**, 648.

WILLIAMS, M., and PENNYBACKER, J. (1954). *J. Neurol. Neurosurg. Psychiat.*, **17**, 115.

CHAPTER 2

THE CARCINOMATOUS NEUROMYOPATHIES

The late Lord Brain, P. B. Croft and Marcia Wilkinson

Recent years have seen considerable advances in our knowledge of the remote effects of cancer on the nervous system. The classification of the resulting phenomena is difficult because it is rarely possible to say more than speculatively how the neoplasm is related to the disorder of function in the nervous system or muscles. The subject has recently been reviewed by Brain and Adams (1965) and their classification will be adopted as a working basis. It is fundamentally a regional classification based on the fact that patients present themselves as clinical problems suffering from lesions which tend predominantly to affect either a particular level of the nervous system or the muscles, though, as will be seen, overlapping is common. Brain and Adams classify these disorders as follows:

CLASSIFICATION OF NON-METASTATIC CARCINOMATOUS NEUROLOGICAL DISEASES

I. Encephalopathy

  1. Multifocal leucoencephalopathy

  2. Diffuse polioencephalopathy
     (a) With mental symptoms
     (b) Subacute cerebellar degeneration
     (c) Brain stem lesions

  3. Encephalopathy due to disordered metabolic or endocrine functions or nutritional deficiency, especially
     (a) Hypercalcæmia with or without bone metastases
     (b) Hyperadrenalism
     (c) Hypoglycæmia
     (d) Hyponatræmia and water intoxication
     (e) Hyperviscosity states especially in macroglobulinæmia

II. Myelopathy

  1. Chronic myelopathy
     (a) Long tract degeneration
     (b) Long tract and neuronal degeneration
     (c) Cases simulating motor neurone disease

    2. Subacute necrotic myelopathy

    3. Nutritional myelopathy

III. Neuropathy

    1. Sensory neuropathy with dorsal column degeneration

    2. Peripheral sensorimotor neuropathy (polyneuropathy or neuritis)

    3. Metabolic, endocrine, and nutritional neuropathies

IV. Muscular Disorders

    1. Polymyopathy

    2. Disorders of neuromuscular transmission
      (a) Myasthenic myopathy with paradoxical potentiation
      (b) Myasthenia gravis

    3. Polymyositis and dermatomyositis

    4. Metabolic myopathies secondary to disordered endocrine function, especially
      (a) Hyperadrenalism
      (b) Hypercalcæmia
      (c) Hyperthyroidism

As we shall see later, multifocal leucoencephalopathy appears on pathological grounds to be distinct from diffuse polioencephalopathy, and the other forms of polioclastic damage to the nervous system which may occur in association with neoplasms. On the other hand the polioclastic type of disorder and the carcinomatous myopathies appear to have some mutual relationship, at least in that they tend to be associated with similar types of neoplasm and with neoplasms which are different from those usually associated with multifocal leucoencephalopathy. For certain statistical purposes, therefore, it has hitherto been the practice to consider the polioclastic type of neuropathy together with the myopathies, under the general heading The Carcinomatous Neuromyopathies.

THE INCIDENCE OF CARCINOMATOUS NEUROMYOPATHY

Croft and Wilkinson (1965) have published a survey of the incidence of carcinomatous neuromyopathy in a large number of men and women with carcinoma at various sites. They acquired their patients in two ways. One group was of unselected patients referred routinely on account of carcinoma, but there was also a group of selected patients who were referred to them because of their known interest in the subject. Table 1 shows the incidence of carcinomatous neuromyopathy discovered:

TABLE 1. INCIDENCE OF CARCINOMATOUS NEUROMYOPATHY

Site of Growth	Males				Females				Total			
	Survey			Selected cases	Survey			Selected cases	Survey			Selected cases
	No. of Patients	Neuromyopathy No.	%		No. of Patients	Neuromyopathy No.	%		No. of Patients	Neuromyopathy No.	%	
Breast	—	—	—	—	250	11	4·4	7	250	11	4·4	7
Lung	247	37	15·0	30	69	8	11·6	10	316	45	14·2	40
Stomach	122	9	7·4	1	56	7	12·5	—	178	16	9·0	1
Colon	61	3	4·9	—	99	3	3·0	1	160	6	3·8	1
Rectum	114	1	0·9	1	93	—	—	—	207	1	0·5	1
Ovary	—	—	—	—	55	9	16·4	2	55	9	16·4	2
Cervix	—	—	—	—	144	3	2·1	—	144	3	2·1	—
Uterus	—	—	—	—	76	1	1·3	1	76	1	1·3	1
Prostate	31	2	6·4	1	—	—	—	—	31	2	6·4	1
Multiple primaries	20	1	5·0	—	28	1	3·6	1	48	2	4·2	1
Miscellaneous primaries	—	—	—	5	—	—	—	6	—	—	—	11
Total	595	53	8·9	38	870	43	4·9	28	1,465	96	6·6	66

TALBE 2. THE INCIDENCE OF SOME DIFFERENT TYPES OF CARCINOMATOUS NEUROMYOPATHY SEEN IN ROUTINE EXAMINATION OF PATIENTS WITH CARCINOMA, AND IN SELECTED PATIENTS REFERRED BECAUSE OF EVIDENCE OF NEUROMYOPATHY

PATIENTS	Cerebellar Degeneration	Myelopathy	Motor Neurone Type	Sensory Neuropathy	Mixed Peripheral Neuropathy	Myopathy Including Myasthenia	Neuro-myopathy	TOTAL
Survey	3 (3%)	3 (3%)	3 (3%)	—	18 (19%)	15 (16%)	62 (65%)	96
Selected	12 (18%)	12 (18%)	8 (12%)	8 (12%)	18 (27%)	11 (17%)	15 (23%)	66
All patients	15 (9%)	15 (9%)	11 (7%)	8 (5%)	36 (22%)	26 (16%)	77 (48%)	162

TYPE OF NEUROMYOPATHY*

* Patients with mixed clinical pictures are included under each relevant heading.

Table 3. Incidence of Some Different Types of Carcinomatous Neuromyopathy in Carcinoma at Various Sites

Site of Carcinoma	Total Patients with Neuromyopathy	Type of Neuromyopathy*						
		Cerebellar	Myelopathy	Motor Neurone Type	Sensory Neuropathy	Mixed Peripheral Neuropathy	Myopathy including Myasthenia	Neuro-myopathy
Breast	18	2 (11%)	1 (6%)	3 (17%)	—	3 (17%)	3 (17%)	8 (44%)
Lung	85	9 (11%)	6 (7%)	5 (6%)	6 (7%)	17 (20%)	17 (20%)	37 (43%)
Stomach	17	—	3 (18%)	2 (12%)	—	5 (29%)	3 (18%)	9 (53%)
Colon	7	—	—	—	1 (14%)	2 (29%)	—	4 (57%)
Rectum	2	—	—	—	—	1 (50%)	—	1 (50%)
Ovary	11	3 (27%)	2 (18%)	—	—	—	2 (18%)	7 (64%)
All other sites combined	22	1 (5%)	3 (14%)	1 (5%)	1 (5%)	8 (36%)	1 (5%)	13 (59%)

* Patients with mixed clinical pictures are included under each relevant heading.

TABLE 4. SITE OF PRIMARY CARCINOMA IN VARIOUS TYPES OF CARCINOMATOUS NEUROMYOPATHY

TYPE OF NEUROMYOPATHY*	TOTAL	SITE OF PRIMARY GROWTH						
		Breast	Lung	Stomach	Colon	Rectum	Ovary	All other Sites Combined
Cerebellar degeneration	15	2 (13%)	9 (60%)	—	—	—	3 (20%)	1 (7%)
Myelopathy	15	1 (7%)	6 (40%)	3 (20%)	—	—	2 (13%)	3 (20%)
Motor neurone type	11	3 (27%)	5 (45%)	2 (18%)	—	—	—	1 (9%)
Sensory neuropathy	8	—	6 (75%)	—	1 (13%)	—	—	1 (13%)
Mixed peripheral neuropathy	36	3 (8%)	17 (47%)	5 (14%)	2 (6%)	1 (3%)	—	8 (22%)
Myopathy including myasthenia and dermatomyositis	26	3 (12%)	17 (65%)	3 (12%)	—	—	2 (8%)	1 (4%)
Neuromuscular	77	8 (10%)	37 (48%)	9 (12%)	4 (5%)	1 (1%)	7 (9%)	11 (14%)
All types	162	18 (11%)	85 (52%)	17 (10%)	7 (4%)	2 (1%)	11 (7%)	22 (14%)

* Patients with mixed clinical pictures are included under each relevant heading.

Table 2 gives the different types of carcinomatous neuro-myopathy in their two series of patients, while Table 3 shows the incidence of the various forms of neuropathy. Table 4 indicates the site of the primary carcinoma in various types of neuro-myopathy.

Croft and Wilkinson explain that they use the term neuromuscular disorder because of the difficulty on clinical grounds alone of distinguishing minor manifestations of a lower motor neurone lesion from minor degrees of a myopathy.

Their figures show that lung carcinoma is responsible for over 50 per cent of all patients seen with evidence of neuromyopathy and that evidence of neuromyopathy is found in 14·2 per cent of all patients with lung carcinoma routinely examined, and in 4·4 per cent of all patients with breast carcinoma. The neuromuscular type of disturbance accounted for approximately 50 per cent of the types of neuromyopathy encountered irrespective of the site of the primary growth. Cerebellar dysfunction was present in 27 per cent of the cases of neuromyopathy in carcinoma of the ovary, and 11 per cent of cases of neuropathy in carcinoma of the breast and lung. Primary myopathic disturbances with or without myasthenia accounted for 17–20 per cent of the cases of neuromyopathy with carcinoma of the breast, lung, or stomach.

THE ASSOCIATION OF NEUROMYOPATHY
WITH DIFFERENT TYPES OF LUNG CARCINOMA

Dayan, Croft and Wilkinson (1965) have studied the incidence of carcinomatous neuromyopathy in relation to different histological types of lung carcinoma. In 37 cases of neuromyopathy associated with carcinoma of the lung the histological type of carcinoma was analysed and compared with that found in 120 cases of carcinoma of the lung without a neuromyopathy and with a further group of 771 patients representative of general hospital experience.

The cases of carcinomatous neuromyopathy showed a preponderance of oat-cell carcinomas and of female patients when compared with both control groups, but the numbers were too small for statistical analysis. There was a suggestive association between the presence of an oat-cell carcinoma and the occurrence of a sensory neuropathy or encephalomyelitic form of neuromyopathy. Similar correlations have been found in 47 cases of carcinomatous neuromyopathy previously reported.

MULTIFOCAL LEUCOENCEPHALOPATHY

This condition was first described by Aström, Mancall and Richardson (1958) and Cavanagh, Greenbaum, Marshall and Rubinstein (1959), and has recently been reviewed by Richardson (1965).

Pathology

The disorder, Richardson points out, is characterized by the occurrence of widely-disseminated lesions of the central nervous system which are demyelinating in that there is total disappearance of myelin sheaths with relative preservation of axis cylinders, and break-down of the myelin into sudanophilic lipids which are contained in the cytoplasm of cerebral macrophages. The lesions vary in size from the microscopic or barely visible to the naked eye, to massive foci involving large parts of a cerebral hemisphere. Although in most cases lesions are most numerous and extensive in the cerebral hemispheres, the brain stem and cerebellum may be severely affected. Typical though sparse lesions have also been found in the spinal cord. In the most advanced cases, the axis cylinders are found to be destroyed also. It has been pointed out that although the disorder is called a leucoencephalopathy, the grey matter may suffer as well as the white.

A remarkable feature of the pathology is the changes in the astrocytes. The astrocytes in the lesions are often gigantic with bizarre deformation of the nucleus, and occasionally contain unequivocal mitotic figures, changes which otherwise occur only in malignant glial tumours. These astrocytic changes, however, are not present in every case, occurring in only 81 per cent of the 44 cases known to Richardson. All the cases, however, have shown a distinctive abnormality of the oligodendrocytes. Those at the periphery of the demyelinated areas show a characteristic enlargement of the nuclei with loss of nuclear detail and inclusion bodies within the nucleus.

Richardson adds that there are no changes in the form or content of the blood vessels which might suggest an ischæmic or angiopathic basis for the cerebral lesions. Also in a large proportion of cases, the cellular phenomena of inflammation in the form of perivascular lymphocytes and plasma cells are lacking. In the others, more or less extensive inflammatory cellular exudates are seen. The absence of such changes, he points out, clearly distinguish this disorder from the large group of multifocal demyelinating encephalopathies represented by post-infectious encephalomyelitis and acute multiple sclerosis in which cellular infiltrations dominate the pathological picture.

Ætiology

Multifocal leucoencephalopathy occurs as a terminal event in a wide range of disorders, most of which involve the reticular system or the blood-forming organs. In the series reviewed by Richardson, in 20 out of 44 cases the patient had chronic lymphocytic leukæmia, Hodgkin's disease, or lymphosarcoma, and there were four cases of myelocytic leukæmia. Among the non-neoplastic reticuloendothelioses were five cases of sarcoidosis and three of tuberculosis, one patient having both, and also three cases of carcinomatosis and a few miscellaneous conditions. These facts led to speculation that multifocal leucoencephalopathy might be due to infection, probably with a virus, secondary to a failure of the usual immune response resulting from the primary disorder from which the patient is suffering. This view now appears to have been confirmed. Zu Rhein and Chou (1965) examining post-mortem tissue fixed in formalin under the electron microscope, found abundant spherical particles exclusively within the nuclei of the oligodendrocytes and in some nuclei there were crystalline organizations of similar particles and elongated cylindrical structures resembling those occasionally seen in cells infected with polyoma virus. Silverman and Rubinstein (1965) have confirmed this observation and Howatson et al. (1965) have provided suggestive evidence that the changes described are due to infection with the polyoma virus. If this view is correct, it would explain two of the pathological features described above (*Lancet* Leader, 1966). The selective demyelination of the early lesions could be attributed to involvement of the oligodendroglia, with important implications for our understanding of other demyelinated disorders. The gross abnormalities in the nuclei of the astrocytes could be understood in the light of the capacity of the polyoma virus to endow the cells which it invades with malignant characteristics.

Clinical Features

Multifocal leucoencephalopathy has hitherto been an invariably fatal disease, running a progressive course lasting from 3–6 months on the average. As the result of the widespread dissemination and variable site of the lesions in the nervous system, the symptomatology is varied. There may be hemiparesis or quadriparesis, visual field defects or even blindness, confusional states, dementia, and aphasia, all the result of lesions of the cerebral hemispheres. If the cerebellum is predominantly involved, the patient will exhibit ataxia and dysarthria. Convulsions are rare. The disorder terminates in coma.

The cerebrospinal fluid is reported usually to be normal. The results of other diagnostic tests are what might be expected from a diffuse cerebral lesion which is not space-occupying.

DIFFUSE POLIOENCEPHALOPATHY

This title best describes a group of patients with a similar pathological picture. The pathological changes tend to be fairly widespread throughout the nervous system but the damage may fall predominantly upon one region, as a result of which a variety of clinical pictures emerge. The subject has recently been reviewed by Henson, Hoffman and Urich (1965), who report five new cases. Adding these to five previously reported cases, they find that the tumour present was in eight instances an oat-cell carcinoma of the bronchus, in one a polygonal cell carcinoma of the breast, and in one an adenocarcinoma of the body of the uterus.

They classify the lesions found in the nervous system into the following groups.

1. Limbic encephalitis, affecting mainly the hippocampal formation, the amygdaloid nucleus, and cingulate and orbital cortex.

2. Bulbar encephalitis, involving mainly the lower brain stem.

3. Myelitis, damaging largely the anterior horn cells at varying levels, and also affecting other cell groups in some instances.

4. Ganglioradiculitis destroying the posterior root ganglia, and causing Wallerian degeneration in the posterior columns and peripheral nerves. Henson *et al.* point out that lesions were generally found in more than one of these four sites.

Pathology

The essential pathological features consist of neuronal destruction and inflammatory infiltration, both diffuse and perivascular, the degeneration and inflammatory infiltration occurring together in varying proportions.

Limbic Encephalitis. In the cases thus classified the lesions have been found to be most severe in the hippocampal formation and amygdaloid nuclei, slightly less marked in the cingulate and orbital cortex, and scanty in other parts of the hemispheres.

Bulbar Encephalitis has been present in 8 of the 10 cases reviewed by Henson *et al.* The inflammatory changes were found predominantly in the lower pons and the medulla, the parts most severely affected being the nuclei in the floor of the 4th ventricle and the inferior olives.

Subacute Cerebellar Degeneration. The pathology of this syndrome is reviewed with the addition of six new cases by Brain and Wilkinson (1965). Loss of Purkinje cells is always a striking feature and in some cases, none can be found. This degeneration is always diffuse. The molecular layer is usually thinner than normal and microglial proliferation has been observed in it. The granular layer may also be narrower than normal and the granule cells sparse. The olives are usually normal. Degeneration of the long tracts of the spinal cord has been observed in a number of cases. In the new cases reported by Brain and Wilkinson, other features included symmetrical areas of degeneration with partial demyelination in the superior cerebellar peduncles, and inflammatory changes in the sub-thalamic nuclei as well as degenerative changes in the brain stem nuclei, and inflammatory changes and partial demyelination of the white matter of the spinal cord.

All these pathological studies show that we are dealing with a diffuse process which may attack all or any levels of the nervous system.

Clinical Features

Onset with Mental Symptoms. In many cases of encephalopathy associated with neoplasm, the onset of symptoms is insidious, and the initial ones may cover a wide range of psychiatric disorders which may lead to the admission of the patient to a mental hospital. These include a simple dementia, which is fairly rapid and progressive, or a disorder of memory, with or without confusion and disorientation. The latter is particularly likely when the pathological changes predominantly involve the limbic areas. On the other hand, the symptoms may be those of a mood disorder such as depression, anxiety, or agitation, with a less prominent disorder of cognition. Psychiatric symptoms may or may not be associated with symptoms and signs of focal cerebral lesions. These latter may also occur with little or no evidence of mental disturbance.

Symptoms of Brain Stem Involvement. These vary according to the distribution of the lesions, ranging from ophthalmoplegia to bulbar palsy, often with nystagmus, ataxia, sometimes involuntary movements, and evidence of bilateral pyramidal tract damage.

Subacute Cerebellar Degeneration. The symptomatology of this has been reviewed by Brain and Wilkinson (1965). The onset is usually subacute. Ataxia was present in all their 19 patients and in

17 in both upper and lower limbs, and dysarthria was p:
14 cases. Nystagmus, however, was absent in more tha
Dysphagia and mental changes were present in 11. There
tendency for the tendon reflexes to be diminished or lost ;
plantar reflexes were either extensor or equivocal in 12 cases

MYELOPATHY

Subacute Necrotic Myelopathy

Mancall and Rosales (1964) have reported two cases and revie ,,ca'
the literature of a condition which they describe as necrotizing
myelopathy associated with visceral carcinoma. This rare disorder
appears to be, both clinically and pathologically, distinct from other
types of neuropathy associated with malignant disease. Clinically,
say Mancall and Rosales, subacute necrotic myelopathy is " characterized by a progressive ascending segmental sensorimotor deficit,
abrupt in onset and rapid in evolution, terminating in death in a
matter of days or weeks. Pathologically, a patchy and non-systematized but roughly symmetrical process of subtotal or total tissue
necrosis involving both grey and white matter has been described;
in most cases the thoracic cord has been particularly severely affected."
In one of their two cases almost the entire spinal cord was involved,
in the other, the changes were almost entirely confined to the mid-
thoracic segments. The basic change was a non-systematized and
patchy, but symmetrical process of destruction of both white and
grey matter in the spinal cord. In the white matter, both myelin
sheaths and axis cylinders were affected, approximately equally.
When the lesions involved grey matter directly the nerve cells were
destroyed. Alterations in the blood vessels were noteworthy. In one
case there was adventitial thickening and fibrosis and frank necrosis,
and in the other only necrosis. These changes involved particularly
small arteries and arterials rather than veins.

The patient develops paraplegia with some impairment of sensibility and loss of sphincter control. The cerebrospinal fluid may be
normal, but more frequently, there is a rise of protein and there may
be an excess of cells, either mononuclear or polymorphs.

Nine similar cases have been found in the literature. The myelopathy was associated with a carcinoma in ten out of the eleven cases:
in the remaining one there was a giant-celled sarcoma. We have seen
a clinically similar case associated with a reticulum-cell sarcoma.

The cause of subacute necrotic myelopathy, like that of other
non-metastatic neurological complications of neoplasms, remains

disease. Although both clinically and pathologically it differs from that of the other forms of neuromyopathy, it is noteworthy that in a few of Mancall and Rosales' cases there were also changes in the muscles characteristic of polymyositis or carcinomatous myopathy.

Motor Neurone Disease

Pathology. The changes in the spinal cord have been described by Norris and Engel (1965) and Brain, Croft and Wilkinson (1965). In the two cases of Brain, Croft and Wilkinson which came to post mortem there was involvement of the lower motor neurone with cell loss in the anterior horns, fibre loss in the anterior roots and peripheral nerves, and denervation atrophy of the skeletal muscles. The authors state that these pathological lesions resembled those seen in motor neurone disease although the changes were less marked than those usually found in the classical form. Moreover both patients showed in addition changes in the posterior root ganglia and posterior columns.

Clinical Features. The symptoms here are those of motor neurone disease or amyotrophic lateral sclerosis. The patient may present with symptoms of bulbar palsy, weakness of one or both upper limbs, or of the lower limbs, or of generalized weakness and lassitude. The signs are those of motor neurone disease with wasting and fasciculation. The tendon reflexes may be exaggerated or diminished, and the plantar reflexes may be flexor or extensor. The course may be more benign and self-limiting than that of motor neurone disease.

Ganglioradiculitis (Sensory Neuropathy)

Pathology. The pathological changes in the posterior root ganglia have been described by Henson *et al.* (1965) and by Croft, Henson, Urich and Wilkinson (1965). The latter authors report four cases of sensory neuropathy associated with bronchial carcinoma. In these cases the pathological changes fell into two groups: sensory neuropathy with Wallerian degeneration of the posterior columns, and scattered inflammatory lesions in the brain and spinal cord. In the posterior root ganglia a large number of nerve cells were destroyed, many being replaced by residual nodules of pyknotic capsule cells. In addition, a small number of cells showed active degenerative changes and sparse lymphocytic infiltration was also present. Similar pathological changes were observed by Henson *et al.* in their series of cases of encephalomyelitis.

Clinical Features. The onset of this is usually subacute, the condition progressing over a period of a few months. Subsequently, the neurological condition often remains unchanged for the duration of the illness which may be as long as twenty months. The striking feature is the sensory disorder, which tends to involve all modes of sensation in both upper and lower limbs, and is often accompanied by distressing paræsthesiæ. There is sensory ataxia and the tendon reflexes are likely to be diminished or lost. Muscular wasting and weakness may also be present. The cerebrospinal fluid frequently shows a rise in protein content, especially in the early stages.

PERIPHERAL SENSORIMOTOR NEUROPATHY
(Polyneuropathy)

Croft, Urich and Wilkinson (1967) have recently published a study of the sensorimotor type of peripheral neuropathy associated with malignant disease. They report 33 patients with this type of disorder, on 10 of whom full neuropathological studies were made. They divide their patients into three groups based on the clinical course of the neurological disorder. These are:

1. Mild and often terminal peripheral neuropathy occurring in the course of known malignant disease.

2. Subacute or acute severe peripheral neuropathy, often occurring before any evidence of malignant disease is present.

3. Patients similar to those in the second group but in whom the neuropathy follows a remitting or sometimes relapsing course. The symptoms are those of a typical polyneuropathy with distal weakness, wasting and sensory loss and diminution or loss of tendon reflexes.

In all their patients studied pathologically the peripheral nerves showed a variable degree of loss of axons and loss of myelin sheaths usually in excess of the damage of the axons. Teased preparations of nerves obtained from two patients confirmed segmental demyelination. Sparse lymphocytic infiltration of peripheral nerves was seen in three cases. The authors suggest that the peripheral neuropathy associated with carcinoma is primarily a demyelinating condition due to disease of Schwann cells with secondary damage to axons.

Hildebrand and Coërs (1967) have recently published a study which contributes to our understanding of some cases of polyneuropathy associated with malignant disease. They studied 46 patients with neoplasms in various sites. Milder symptoms of peripheral motor neuropathy were found in two emaciated patients. In 14 others, the muscle wasting and occasional weakness were diffuse and not suggestive of a specific neuromuscular disorder. The only consistent electromyographic change was post-tetanic facilitation in 4 patients, most marked in weak and wasted muscles in two instances. No significant reduction of conduction velocity in motor nerves was obtained in any patient. The histological changes found were an increased collateral branching of motor nerve fibres and abnormal volumetric variations of the muscle fibres. These changes, indicating a subclinical involvement of peripheral nerves, were observed in 5 of 11 patients who had recently lost weight, without any actual emaciation or cachexia and in 12 of the 16 emaciated patients. Thus histological abnormalities of the neuropathic type were present in 17 of the 27 patients with clinical evidence of malnutrition. The authors stress this association in relation to the possible ætiology of carcinomatous neuromuscular disorders.

Cerebrospinal Fluid. In Croft, Urich and Wilkinson's series, the changes in the cerebrospinal fluid were similar to those found in patients in whom the central nervous system is involved. The cell count is usually normal. The protein content exceeded 100 mg/100 ml in 8 patients and 120 mg/100 ml in 7, the highest figure recorded being 360 mg/100 ml. Changes in the colloidal gold curve were fairly frequently found and 3 patients had a curve of the paretic type.

Electrodiagnostic Tests. Electrodiagnostic tests in the same series yielded varied results. In some cases there was evidence of a sensori-motor neuropathy, in others, the motor conduction velocities were markedly reduced, and in two cases there was also electrical evidence of a myopathic disturbance.

THE NEUROMYOPATHIES

Some clarification of terms is necessary to begin with. The term "neuromyopathy" has been used comprehensively to include all the disorders of the central and peripheral nervous system and muscles which may be remote effects of malignant disease. It has also been used in a narrower sense by Croft and Wilkinson (1963) to denote a group of cases in which it is impossible to say on clinical grounds alone whether the disorder is primarily muscular or secondary to neural degeneration, or both. Shy and Silverstein (1965) retain this as a useful term and define it as follows: "The term 'neuromyopathy' . . . designates a definitive clinical syndrome of symmetrical proximal muscle weakness and wasting, associated with decrease of the appropriate myotatic reflexes. Either a myopathic or a combination of myopathic and neuropathic lesion was noted in the biopsies of all affected individuals."

These neuromyopathies are by far the commonest of the remote effects of malignant disease, constituting 65 per cent of such manifestations seen in the routine examination of patients with carcinoma (Croft and Wilkinson, 1965). In Shy and Silverstein's series of 42 patients comprising those with central and peripheral nervous lesions, as well as disorders of the motor unit, 26 presented with neuromyopathy.

The general features of this syndrome have been described in previous papers (Lennox and Pritchard, 1950). A striking and important feature is that the symptoms of muscular weakness may, and usually do, antedate the symptoms of malignancy, often by several years. As Shy and Silverstein point out, the predominant complaints of all patients are "difficulty in standing, rising from a sitting position, and climbing stairs. The muscles most frequently involved were the deltoids, supraspinatus, triceps, sternocleidomastoids, quadriceps, brachioradialis, glutei, iliopsoas, adductors and hamstrings. All patients had involvement of both sides of the body, 20 were symmetrical, and 6 more on one side than the other. 2 patients had in addition severe fatigue and bulbar involvement . . . 3 patients had dysphagia." The tendon reflexes in affected muscles are diminished or lost.

Mixed pictures are not uncommon. The central nervous system may be involved in one of the varieties described above, as well as the muscles. Mental symptoms may be present. In Shy and Silverstein's series, 4 patients had Raynaud's phenomenon, 3 had skin lesions and 5 transitory and migratory arthropathies, while 3 showed intermittent gross fasciculation.

THE MYOPATHIES

Since carcinomatous neuromyopathy was first described, there has been much discussion about the nature and significance of the pathological changes in the muscles. How, it is asked, are these related to dermatomyositis and polymyositis? On the other hand, it has been questioned whether there are any specific changes in the muscles. These questions have recently been discussed by Rowland and Schotland (1965) and Shy and Silverstein (1965). Shy and Silverstein studied a total of 151 patients that presented with a late onset of symmetrical proximal muscular weakness and wasting, and of whom 27 had malignant disease. They found in both groups of patients pathological changes suggestive of a myopathic lesion, equal amounts of inflammation could be found in both the non-carcinomatous and carcinomatous groups. Aggregates of inflammatory cells were seldom found in the neoplastic group. Both groups of patients demonstrated pathological changes suggestive of a myopathic lesion: i.e. loss of cross-striations, floccular, cloudy and granular changes, and internally placed nuclei with an increase of endomysial connective tissue. Many cases demonstrated basophilic fibres with large vesicular nuclei and prominent nucleoli characteristic of regeneration of muscle.

It would seem that muscles have a very limited number of ways of responding to various noxæ. In a case of proximal myopathy of late onset it may be impossible to distinguish histologically between the carcinomatous and non-carcinomatous group. Whether carcinomatous myopathy is identical with polymyositis as Rose and Walton (1966) appear to believe, must remain unsettled until we understand better the pathogenesis of both.

Electrophysiology. Shy and Silverstein report the results of their investigation of 15 patients with carcinomatous neuromyopathy. All showed evidence of a myopathic lesion in that a normal interference or mixed pattern in the phase of muscle weakness was obtained. In addition, there was a significantly short mean action potential which was derived from 20 different motor units of the muscle samples. Finally there was a marked increase in short polyphasic potentials. 5 patients had in addition evidence of a neuropathic involvement as well.

The Myasthenic Syndrome

The myasthenic syndrome has recently been discussed by Lambert and Rooke (1965) and by Shy and Silverstein (1965). Lambert and Rooke report that out of 30 patients with the myasthenic syndrome 22 had, or subsequently developed, intrathoracic tumours. They had not found a myasthenic syndrome except in patients with carcinoma of the bronchus but other authors have reported the disorder with carcinoma elsewhere. Shy and Silverstein defined the syndrome as "a clinical constellation of weakness and fatigue of both bulbar and somatic musculature. Patients so afflicted may show either facilitation or a reduction of repetitive action potentials obtained upon stimulation of the appropriate nerve to the muscle so recorded. Such patients may or may not respond to anticholinesterases. Unlike patients with myasthenia gravis, these patients commonly exhibit diminution of myotatic reflexes," and, one might add, sometimes muscular wasting also.

The initial symptom, as well as the major complaint in almost all patients, was weakness and easy fatiguability of the legs. Weakness of the arms was less frequently complained of. About a third of the patients reported a transient episode of blurring of vision or ptosis.

Dryness of the mouth was experienced by at least half of the patients and in 2 it was a major complaint. Peripheral paræsthesiæ and loss of sexual potency were reported by almost half the patients. A clinical feature of the weakness was an appreciable delay in the development of strength and the onset of maximal voluntary contraction. This was evident in peripheral muscles, for example in the grip, as well as in the proximal muscles of the extremities. With prolonged exertion weakness developed more rapidly than in normal persons.

Electrophysiological Studies. Lambert and Rooke describe the electromyographic findings which they regard as characteristic of the syndrome. The action potential and the twitch evoked in a rested muscle by a single maximal stimulus are greatly reduced in amplitude even though the strength of voluntary contraction may be normal or nearly so. Repetitive stimulation of the nerve at a slow rate (two shocks per second) produces a further decrease in amplitude of the action potential and twitch which is progressive for the first few responses. However, during stimulation at fast rates (10–200 per second) a progressive increase in response occurs. The increase occurs at rates of stimulation comparable to the rate of impulses in motor neurones during strong voluntary contraction (20–40 per second). Thus, facilitation of the response during repetitive excitation accounts for the fact that strength of voluntary contraction may be normal, even though the strength of a single twitch or arrested muscle is greatly reduced. This phenomenon has been called paradoxical potentiation. Lambert and Rooke discuss its possible mechanism. Shy and Silverstein, however, point out that not all patients with a myasthenic syndrome associated with bronchogenic carcinoma show facilitation. Some exhibit the classical myasthenic-type picture with decrease of the action potential on multiple stimuli. They also point out that a patient may have both a myasthenic syndrome and symmetrical proximal weakness and wasting. Such patients may respond to Tensilon. In the myasthenic syndrome, Tensilon produces some effect but much less than in myasthenia gravis. Patients with either condition may be unduly sensitive to muscle relaxants.

The response of the myasthenic syndrome to the treatment of the neoplasm is extremely variable. Temporary improvement does sometimes follow therapy and we have seen a patient who had a complete remission of the myasthenic syndrome after radiotherapy to a lung carcinoma, only to relapse when the carcinoma began to grow again.

ENDOCRINE DISORDERS ASSOCIATED WITH MALIGNANT DISEASE

Apart from the more purely neurological manifestations produced remotely by various types of malignant disease, endocrine and meta-bolic disturbances may occur in association with neoplasms. These have been described in association with many different types of malignant disease, although as with the neurological disturbances, there is a particular association with oat-cell carcinoma of the bronchus, and include the ectopic ACTH syndrome, hyponatræmic syndrome, hypercalcæmia, hypoglycæmia, the carcinoid syndrome, skin pigmentation, thyrotoxicosis, and gynæcomastia.

The Ectopic ACTH Syndrome. Some patients develop a bio-chemical disturbance resembling Cushing's syndrome and this disorder is now often called the "Ectopic ACTH Syndrome." Like many clinical syndromes, the more assiduously one looks for it the more frequently it will be discovered. In a survey of 100 cases of carcinoma of the lung, adrenal hyperplasia has been found in 2 per cent. While oat-cell carcinoma of the lung is the growth most frequently responsible for this syndrome, it has been reported in patients with malignant disease at many other sites.

These patients do not show the typical clinical stigmata of Cushing's syndrome, probably because they usually die within a few weeks of the syndrome being established. There is much less obesity, osteoporosis and striæ than in typical Cushing's syndrome. The presenting symptoms of the ectopic ACTH syndrome include œdema of the lower limbs, muscular weakness often made worse by diuretics, loss of tendon reflexes, periods of confusion, symptoms of diabetes mellitus including thirst and polyuria, and skin pigmentation.

The essential biochemical disturbance is an increase in circulating ACTH activity, and bioassays have shown such activity to be present in the primary tumour and in metastases, with sub-normal amounts in the pituitary and none at all in non-tumourous tissue. The ACTH-like substance has close similarities to pituitary ACTH but it is quite possible that the active principle may be a polypeptide of smaller size than the normal ACTH molecule. There is hypokalæmic alkalosis with a very high level of circulating cortisol, excessive loss of potassium in the urine, and loss of the normal diurnal cortisol variation. ACTH stimulation tests do not increase the serum cortisol or urinary 17-OHCS levels, presumably because the adrenal cortex is already under maximal stimulation. Dexamethasone suppression tests do not reduce the cortisol level as it does in ordinary Cushing's syndrome, since in the ectopic ACTH syndrome the cortisol output is no longer under pituitary control. Patients have been treated by adrenalectomy, by removal of, or radiotherapy to, the primary tumour.

The muscular weakness shown by these patients may be in part a result of the hypokalæmia and in part a form of steroid myopathy.

Hyponatræmia. This has been described mainly in association with oat-cell carcinoma of the lung, though cases have also occurred in association with tuberculosis and some brain disorders (including head injury, pituitary tumours, vascular disease and encephalitis). The clinical picture is a rather ill-defined one of increasing lethargy, confusion and drowsiness. Biochemically, the most striking abnormality is the hyponatræmia, the serum sodium being as low as 110 mEq per litre. This hyponatræmia is usually mainly of a dilutional type associated with a slightly low serum chloride and normal potassium, a low blood urea (less than 20 mg/100 ml) and a low packed cell volume, the plasma volume being increased. The osmolarity of the urine is greater than that of the plasma. The increased plasma volume reduces aldosterone secretion and hence there is a further loss of sodium so that the hyponatræmia may become partly depletional as well as dilutional. Corresponding to the findings in the ectopic ACTH syndrome in hyponatræmia, antidiuretic (ADH) activity has been demonstrated in tumour tissue, and the syndrome appears to be due to an inappropriate secretion of a substance with ADH activity, this secretion continuing in spite of the dilutional hyponatræmia.

The patients are improved by water restriction and particularly by treatment with 9-α-hydrofluorocortisone. The use of cytoxic drugs to the primary growth has occasionally produced improvement.

Hypercalcæmia. While hypercalcæmia in malignant disease is often due to the presence of bony metastases, it may occur in the absence of such bony deposits, particularly in association with primary carcinoma of the bronchus and hypernephroma. The main symptoms include malaise, thirst, polyuria and polydipsia and later vomiting and coma. A recent paper reported six cases of hypercalcæmia without bony metastases in 100 consecutive cases of bronchial carcinoma (Carey, 1966). The hypercalcæmia can be reversed by treatment with cortisone, and also when possible by removal of the primary tumour. The condition tends to recur if metastases develop later.

In the endocrine disturbances associated with malignant disease there is now good evidence that the tumour may secrete a substance with biochemical activity resembling naturally occurring hormones and sometimes more than one such substance is produced.

Although endocrine and neurological disorders do not frequently occur together in one patient such associations are not unknown. Recently Hallpike and Morgan-Hughes (1966) have reported a patient with bronchial carcinoma who developed hyponatræmia and myasthenia and Sethurajan, Croft and Wilkinson (1967) have reported a case of bronchial neoplasm with endocrine, metabolic and neurological manifestations.

In peripheral sensorimotor neuropathy we have seen disturbances of glucose, sodium and potassium metabolism in individual patients as well as pigmentation due to secretion of melanocyte stimulating hormone (MSH).

It is not necessary to postulate that all of the diverse remote effects produced by carcinoma are the result of a single pathological process. Some may be found to be the result of a specific virus infection, while others have a purely hormonal basis. On the other hand it may be that in cases where a virus is incriminated, the neurological disturbance results from an abnormal response to a commonly occurring virus, the altered response being caused by some polypeptide secreted by the primary tumour.

References

ASTRÖM, K. E., MANCALL, E. L., and RICHARDSON, E. P. (1958). *Brain*, **81**, 93.

BRAIN and ADAMS, R. D. (1965). In *The Remote Effects of Cancer on the Nervous System*, ed. Brain and Norris, F. H., p. 216. New York, Grune & Stratton.

BRAIN and NORRIS, F. H. (1965). *The Remote Effects of Cancer on the Nervous System*, New York, Grune & Stratton.

BRAIN and WILKINSON, M. (1965). *Brain*, **88**, 465.

BRAIN, CROFT, P. B., and WILKINSON, M. (1965). *Brain*, **88**, 479.

CAREY, V. C. (1966). *Amer. Rev. resp. Dis.*, **93**, 584.

CAVANAGH, J. B., GREENBAUM, D., MARSHALL, A. H. E., and RUBINSTEIN, L. J., (1959). *Lancet*, **2**, 524.

CROFT, P. B., and WILKINSON, M. (1963). *Lancet*, **1**, 184.

CROFT, P. B., and WILKINSON, M. (1965). *Brain*, **88**, 427.

CROFT, P. B., HENSON, R. A., URICH, H., and WILKINSON, P. C. (1965). *Brain*, **88**, 501.

CROFT, P. B., URICH, H., and WILKINSON, M. (1967). *Brain*, **90**, 31.

DAYAN, A. D., CROFT, P. B., and WILKINSON, M. (1965). *Brain*, **88**, 435.

HALLPIKE, J. F., and MORGAN-HUGHES, J. A. (1966). *Brit. med. J.*, **2**, 1573.

HENSON, R. A., HOFFMAN, H. L., and URICH, H. (1965). *Brain*, **88**, 449.

HILDEBRAND, J., and COËRS, C. (1967). *Brain*, **90**, 67.

HOWATSON, A. F., NAGAI, M., and ZU RHEIN, G. M. (1965). *Canad. med. Ass. J.*, **93**, 379.

LAMBERT, E. H., and ROOKE, E. D. (1965). In *The Remote effects of Cancer on the Nervous System*, ed. Brain and Norris, F. H., p. 67. New York, Grune & Stratton.

Lancet (1966). Leading article, **1**, 353.

LENNOX, B., and PRITCHARD, S. (1950). *Quart. J. Med.*, **19**, 97.

MANCALL, E. L., and ROSALES, R. K. (1964). *Brain*, **87**, 639.

NORRIS, F. H., and ENGEL, W. K. (1965). In *The Remote Effects of Cancer on the Nervous System*, ed. Brain and Norris, F. H., p. 24. New York, Grune & Stratton.

RICHARDSON, E. P. (1965). In *The Remote Effects of Cancer on the Nervous System*, ed. Brain and Norris, F. H., p. 6, New York, Grune & Stratton.

ROSE, A. L., and WALTON, J. N. (1966). *Brain*, **89**, 747.

ROWLAND, L. P., and SCHOTLAND, D. L. (1965). In *The Remote Effects of Cancer on the Nervous System*, ed. Brain and Norris, F. H., p. 83. New York, Grune & Stratton.

SETHURAJAN, C., CROFT, P. B., and WILKINSON, M. (1967). *Neurology*, **17**, 1169.

SHY, G. M., and SILVERSTEIN, I. (1965). *Brain*, **88**, 515.

SILVERMAN, L., and RUBINSTEIN, L. J. (1965). *Acta neuropath.* **5**, 215.

ZU RHEIN, G. M., and CHOU, S. M. (1965). *Science*, **148**, 1477.

CHAPTER 3

OTONEUROLOGY

The late LORD BRAIN

THE two main lines of advance in otoneurology have been the development of new tests of auditory and vestibular function, or the modification of old tests, and partly as a result of these, the recognition of new syndromes and the better evaluation of old ones. This chapter begins, therefore, with a description of recent advances in methods of investigation.

TESTS OF AUDITORY FUNCTION

Loudness Recruitment Test

The loudness recruitment test is described by Dix (1956) and Hallpike (1965). It is carried out as follows. The subject wears a pair of telephone receivers, each supplied from a separate pure tone generator. The frequency of the sound stimulus is the same in each receiver but its intensity can be adjusted independently, and it is switched alternately to left and right. The subject is asked to say when the sound appears equally loud in the two ears. When one ear is deaf, the intensity of the sound will have to be greater in that ear in order that the sound may appear equally loud in the two ears. The object of the test is to discover whether the relative difference between these two intensities remains the same as the loudness of the sound is increased or not. At one extreme, the difference of intensity remains the same, however much the loudness of the sound is increased: at the other extreme, the more the loudness is increased, the less the difference between the two ears, until in some cases at a certain degree of loudness the stimuli required to produce it are the same in both ears. This is the phenomenon of loudness recruitment.

What is the diagnostic significance of the loudness recruitment test? When the deafness is of the conductive type loudness recruitment is absent. Hallpike reports the results of applying this test in 50 cases of partial unilateral perceptive or nerve deafness, in 30 of which the deafness was due to Ménière's disease, and in 20 to tumours. In all

35

the 30 cases of Ménière's disease, loudness recruitment was found to be present and complete. In 14 of the 20 cases of 8th nerve tumour, recruitment was absent, and in the remaining six cases it was present but incomplete. These findings have subsequently been confirmed by further studies.

Hallpike concludes that loudness recruitment is characteristically present in a disorder of the cochlear end organs, and is absent in a disorder of the cochlear nerve fibres. It is valuable, therefore, in discriminating between these two categories of perceptive deafness. Hallpike quotes a recent study by Dix on nerve deafness in multiple sclerosis in which loudness recruitment is characteristically absent. Hallpike concludes that loudness recruitment is characteristic of a lesion of the cochlear hair cells, in inner ear disease, because that leads to a selective destruction of the low intensity elements which results in deafness, while the high intensity elements are preserved and hence good loudness is produced at high intensity levels. When, however, the lesion involves the fibres from these cells, either in the 8th nerve itself or between its point of entry to the pons and the cochlear nucleus, the fibre degeneration is evenly distributed, and therefore affects both low and high intensity fibres alike, and since there is no selective sparing of either, loudness recruitment is absent in 90 per cent of cases of nerve fibre deafness.

Other Audiometric Tests

A number of further tests or refinements of existing ones have been introduced with the object of providing more information about the cochlea and the auditory pathways in the nervous system.

Speech Test

The hearing of spoken words is a highly complex process. The auditory stimulus covers a wide range of frequencies transformed by the cochlea into on-off impulses carried by a wide range of nerve fibres in the auditory nerve. A lesion of this nerve may leave intact enough fibres to convey a considerable amount of information about pure tones at certain frequencies, but it is bound to disturb the complex interrelationships of impulses upon which the hearing of spoken speech depends.

The examiner, who should not be visible to the patient, pronounces a series of familiar two-syllable words which depend for their recognition largely on vowel sounds, and then a series of one-syllable words which are recognized mainly by their higher pitched consonants. Fifty such words are given, representing a total score of a hundred. A score of 40 per cent to 80 per cent indicates cochlear damage. In Ménière's disease during a remission in the earlier stages, speech discrimination may be normal or nearly so. Later it tends to fluctuate from time to time. In cases of acoustic neuroma, speech discrimination is always low. In a series of 45 cases of acoustic neuroma nearly 70 per cent achieved a discrimination score of 30 per cent or less (Johnson and House, 1964).

Békésy Audiometry

Békésy audiometry is a refined technique whereby the patient records his own threshold automatically over the whole range of frequencies (von Békésy, 1947). The test begins with the introduction into the earphone of a pure tone of very low frequency below the patient's threshold for loudness. The tone gradually becomes louder and the patient is instructed to press a button as soon as he hears it. The tone then gradually becomes fainter and he is instructed to press the button again when he ceases to hear it. This process continues with the tone gradually increasing in frequency, and the behaviour of the tone and the patient's interruptions are recorded. Two such tracings are made on each ear, one with a continuous pure tone and the other with a pure tone which is turned on and off rapidly, and is therefore called an interrupted tone. The two traces are made with differently coloured inks. Jerger (1960) classifies Békésy audiometry tracings into five types. In Type I the records for continuous and interrupted tones are superimposed. This type occurs with normal hearing and with a conductive deafness. In the Type II curve, the two tracings are superimposed up to about 1,000 CPS and above this, the continuous tone tracing falls below the interrupted tone tracing, but never more than 30 db, owing to end-organ fatigue. Furthermore, the interrupted tracing shows a narrow amplitude at higher frequencies indicating recruitment. This type of curve is characteristic of cochlear disorders. In the Type III audiogram the curve for the interrupted tone behaves normally but that for the continuous tone falls away sharply and progressively as the frequency increases. In the Type IV audiogram the curve for the continuous tone falls below that for the interrupted tone at all frequencies. The significance of these tracings is discussed by Johnson and House (1964) who point out that the differentiation between a Type II and Type IV tracing may be difficult. In their series of acoustic neuromas, 40 per cent of cases exhibited a Type IV pattern and the next most common tracing was Type III, the two together constituting 70 per cent, but in the remainder of cases of surgically confirmed neuromas, Type I or Type II tracings occurred. In Type V the continuous tracing is better than the interrupted one. This is usually obtained in psychogenic deafness, but is not conclusive evidence of this.

Tone Decay Test (Synonyn-Adaptation)

This test is similar to the Békésy continuous tone test except that only a conventional audiometer is required (Rosenberg, 1958, Green, 1963). A continuous tone of 5 db above threshold is introduced and as soon as the subject indicates that it is no longer heard, the intensity is increased 5 db. This is continued for 60 seconds. As in the Békésy test, a diseased cochlea shows fatigue to the continuous tone which is manifested by the number of times the increment must be added. When the patient has a normal or only a slightly depressed cochlea, it is necessary to add from 0 to 15 db in the 60 seconds. When the cochlea is more severely depressed, 15 to 30 db must be added in 5 db increments. If it is necessary to add more than 30 db it is suggestive of 8th nerve involvement.

The SISI Test

The SISI (Short Increment Sensitivity Index) test (Jerger, Shedd and Harford, 1959) consists of presenting to the patient a steady tone 20 db above threshold for 2 minutes. Every 5 seconds the intensity jumps 1 db for 2/10ths of a second, and if the patient hears the jump, he pushes a button. After 20 such increments, the number of times the patient has pushed the button is counted and the final score is the percentage of the 20 increments that were heard. This procedure is carried out at different frequencies. This test is chiefly of value in differentiating cochlear disorders from others. When the disorder is in the cochlea the patient will be able to hear very small changes in intensity and is likely to score from 50–100 per cent in frequencies above 1,000 cps, whereas patients with middle ear lesions or with 8th nerve disorders ordinarily score from 0–20 per cent at all frequencies.

Summary of Characteristic Test Results with Lesions in Different Situations

Site of Lesion	SISI	Békésey Type	Loudness Recruitment
Middle ear	−	I	Absent
Cochlear	+	II	Partial or complete
8th nerve	−	III or IV	Absent or partial

CALORIC TESTS

Electronystagmography

Electronystagmography is a method of recording nystagmus described by Aschan and Stahle (1956). The patient is placed in the recumbent position with the head elevated 30° to place the horizontal semicircular canal in a position for maximum stimulation. An electrode is applied lateral to each eye with a ground electrode in the centre of the forehead to record horizontal nystagmus. Electrodes are placed above and below one eye to record vertical nystagmus. The movements of the eye which occur with nystagmus cause the differential in potential between the cornea and the retina to be displaced laterally, which leads to a recordable change in potential at the outer canthus. Electronystagmography makes it possible to record the precise moment of onset and the duration of the nystagmus, the maximum frequency, amplitude, and speed of beat. It also makes recording possible in various positions of the head and with the eyes open or closed.

Directional Preponderance

The concept of directional preponderance is not new, but it is so important in relation to vestibular testing that a summary of its significance will be given based upon a recent paper by Hallpike (1965). The caloric test is carried out in the usual way and the result recorded as shown in Fig. 2 as the results of testing the left and right ears with water at a temperature of 30°C and 44°C. These responses are numbered from 1–4 from above downwards, and it will be seen that responses 1 and 4 consist of nystagmus to the right, responses 2 and 3 of nystagmus to the left, the direction of the nystagmus being specified in terms of its rapid component in accordance with convention.

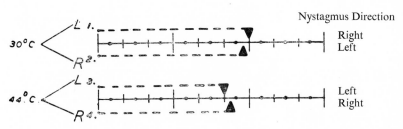

Figure 2. Caloric Test: normal.

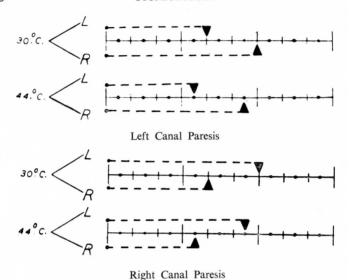

Figure 3. Caloric Tests: left canal paresis and right canal paresis.

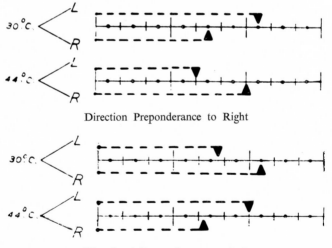

Figure 4. Caloric Tests: directional preponderance.

(Figs. 2–4 reproduced from Fitzgerald and Hallpike (1942) by kind permission.)

Hallpike points out that two primary abnormalities of this pattern may be produced by a unilateral vestibular lesion. The commonest of these is the reduction of sensitivity of one or other canal—the so-called canal paresis. This is shown in Fig. 3 above. With a left canal paresis responses 1 and 3 are reduced compared with responses 2 and 4 which are normal; below with a right canal paresis, this pattern is reversed.

However, another type of abnormality, known as directional preponderance may occur. Directional preponderance means that those responses which consist of nystagmus in a particular direction are facilitated with inhibition of their opposites. As shown in Fig. 4 with directional preponderance (DP) to the right, responses 1 and 4, which consist of nystagmus to the right, are increased, while responses 2 and 3 are decreased. With DP to the left, this pattern is reversed. Directional preponderance is systematically directed towards the side opposite to the lesion which causes it. Thus, a left-sided lesion causes preponderance to the right, and vice versa.

Hallpike observes that one or other of these abnormal responses may be necountered in association with a unilateral vestibular lesion at any level between the labyrinth and the vestibular nuclei. Usually they occur separately: they may, however, be combined, in which case the resulting caloric test pattern represents an algebraic summation of the two primary abnormalities.

Hallpike argues that since a unilateral vestibular lesion may result in either one of these two abnormalities, they must depend upon damage to elements which are anatomically separate. In canal paresis, the lesion involves one of the cupular sense organs or their associated nerve fibres, or nuclei. In the case of directional preponderance, it is postulated that the lesion involves one of the tonus organs of the labyrinth, in particular the utricle, or its associated neurones in the vestibular nerve or nuclei.

Carmichael, Dix and Hallpike (1965) have reported a study of directional preponderance in 8 subjects who exhibited the symptoms and signs of unilateral lesions due to arterial occlusion of the lateral zone of the medulla. All these patients showed evidence of organic vestibular disturbance including directional preponderance to the side opposite to the lesion. The sites and extents of the lesions were determined by means of close analysis of the neurological abnormalities, and plotted upon a series of brainstem sections. This established the relationship of the lesions to the vestibular nuclear complex, and identified the nuclei most likely to have been damaged. The damage was found to be limited to the most caudal of the vestibular nuclei, i.e. the descending nucleus and the caudal part of the medial nucleus. Directional preponderance was therefore attributed to organic damage of these nuclei.

The interpretation of directional preponderance offered is as follows. The vestibular tonus elements, left and right, exert a pair of forces, opposed and balanced upon the conjugate deviation of the eyes. The left elements subserve deviation to the right, and the right elements to the left. If, therefore, the left elements are damaged, there will be a latent deviation of the eyes to the left, and conversely. Nystagmus of the vestibular type, whether spontaneous or induced, is increased if the gaze be voluntarily deviated from its normal resting position in the direction of the nystagmus, while gaze deviation in the opposite direction will reduce the nystagmus.

The Minimal Caloric Test

The modification of the caloric test has been introduced by Pulec, House and Hughes (1964). It is known as the Linthicum or Minimal Caloric Test, and its object is to simplify the procedure and minimize discomfort to the patient. The patient is seated with his elbow resting on the arm of the chair, the head is placed on the hand so that the ear to be tested is uppermost. 0·2 ml of iced water is instilled into the external auditory meatus and allowed to remain there for 20 seconds. The head is then tilted to the opposite side so that the water may drain out of the ear canal. The patient is then instructed to look at a spot on the ceiling with the head tipped back 60°. A small scleral blood vessel is observed to determine whether there is a horizontal nystagmus present. The head is then tilted forward at an angle of 30° and the scleral blood vessel is observed for rotary nystagmus. If the vertigo induced troubles the patient, 0·2 ml of warm water may be instilled into the ear to neutralize the cold. Should the patient fail to respond to 0·2 ml, 0·4 ml is used and then 0·8 ml and finally, 2 ml. If there is no response to 2 ml the ear is considered to be non-reactive. A time of approximately 5 minutes should be allowed to elapse between the test of the first and the second ear. This is a much simpler version of the usual caloric test and may be applicable in circumstances in which the usual procedure cannot be carried out. It cannot however be used to demonstrate directional preponderance. The ordinary test is to be preferred when possible.

We will now consider the application of these diagnostic methods to the recognition of new syndromes and the interpretation of old ones.

MÉNIÈRES DISEASE

The cardinal clinical features of Ménière's Disease have long been recognized and need not here be described in detail. The cause of Ménière's Disease is now generally recognized to be endolymphatic distension of the labyrinth, though why this occurs is uncertain. The cardinal symptoms are paroxysmal vertigo accompanied by nausea and vomiting, deafness, and tinnitus. Hallpike (1955) reports the result of caloric tests in 100 cases of Ménière's Disease. There was canal paresis in 49 cases and directional preponderance in 21. The two were present together in 18 cases and 12 patients gave normal responses. Loudness recruitment is always present.

The treatment of Ménière's Disease is described below.

VESTIBULAR NEURONITIS

The term "vestibular neuronitis" was introduced by Dix and Hallpike (1952). Vestibular neuronitis differs from Ménière's Disease in the absence of cochlear symptoms and signs. It may affect either adults or children and is relatively more common than Ménière's Disease under the age of 30. The vertigo may resemble that of Ménière's Disease, or may consist of sudden seizures accompanied by sensations of blackout, or there may be simply a feeling of unsteadiness and lack of balance when walking. The onset of symptoms is not uncommonly associated with those of some kind of febrile illness.

Tests of cochlear function show no abnormality. Caloric tests, however, constantly show severe and often bilateral derangement. Involvement of the vestibular fibres with sparing of the cochlear ones locates the lesion central to the labyrinth and it has been thought to be the result of damage to the vestibular fibres within the brain stem, presumably by some toxic or inflammatory process.

The condition is usually a benign one, improvement gradually occurring both in the symptoms and the caloric responses.

BENIGN POSITIONAL VERTIGO

The precipitation of vertigo by changes in the position of the head has been recognized for many years. We owe to Dix and Hallpike (1952) the isolation of the benign form, so-called because it is not a symptom of any serious intracranial disease. The condition chiefly affects adults for the age group 30–60 years, and the onset is commonly acute. The characteristic feature of the disorder is the mode of eliciting the vertigo and accompanying nystagmus. The patient sits upon a couch with the head turned either to the right or to the left. The examiner then grasps the patient's head and pushes him back into the supine position with the head extended as well as rotated to the side. After a latent interval of a few seconds, the patient experiences vertigo and some distress and nystagmus appears, chiefly rotatary, the direction of the rotation being towards the undermost ear. In addition, there is generally a horizontal component, also directed towards the undermost ear. The nystagmus increases for some seconds and then rapidly declines, the patient at the same time feeling more comfortable. If the procedure is repeated two or three times in rapid succession the nystagmus diminishes and finally disappears, and cannot be elicited again until after a period of rest.

Dix and Hallpike concluded that the symptoms were due to an irritative lesion of the otolith apparatus of the labyrinth towards which, when undermost, the nystagmus was directed. The evidence for this was the benign course of the disease and the absence of evidence of any involvement of the central nervous system, and a labyrinthine lesion was indicated by the fact that in 55 of their 100 cases, substantial evidence of ear disease was present, usually in the form of gross middle ear infection or labyrinthine trauma. In one typical case a histological examination of the affected labyrinth revealed chronic changes in the otolith apparatus.

The prognosis of benign positional vertigo is usually good, but the symptoms may recur.

ACOUSTIC NEUROMA

It is useful, following Hallpike, to distinguish two distinct stages in the evolution of an acoustic neuroma. In the first, or otological stage, there is a slow and progressive destruction of both cochlear and vestibular nerve fibres. The deafness is, of course, unilateral, and it is usually accompanied by tinnitus which is not often severe. Vertigo is slight in the early stages and amounts to little more than unsteadiness and momentary giddiness on walking. As the tumour expands from the internal auditory meatus, it enters the neurological stage, pressing upon the brain stem, and later, the cerebellum, and finally causing symptoms and signs of increased intracranial pressure. The aim of diagnosis should be the detection of the tumour in its first, otological, stage, which means the complete investigation of every patient suffering from unilateral deafness, however slight.

Audiometric Tests

The results of audiometric tests in 55 cases of acoustic neuroma have recently been reviewed by Johnson and House (1964). High tone loss was present in 67 per cent of cases and severe impairment of speech discrimination in about 69 per cent. Békésy audiometry in the majority of cases yielded a Type III or Type IV response. The Sisi test score was more often low than high. The authors draw attention to the large group of cases with inconsistent auditory findings. Loudness recruitment is usually absent, but when it is present it is always incomplete.

Vestibular Tests

Tests of vestibular function always give abnormal results. The commonest abnormality is canal paresis, which may occur in combination with a directional preponderance to the unaffected side. Occasionally the latter abnormality is present alone.

Neurological Signs

When the tumour is at the otological stage, there will be no neurological signs, as a rule, though the facial nerve lies in close relationship with the tumour in the internal auditory canal. Special tests designed to detect minimal degrees of facial nerve involvement have been carried out by Pulec and House (1964). These include a test for delay in the blink reflex, detection of impairment of taste on the anterior two-thirds of the tongue by means of an electric taste-detector, and a comparison of the secretion of tears on the two sides. Attention has also been drawn to hypæsthesia of the posterior aspect of the external auditory canal, which is said to be present in a high proportion of acoustic neuroma cases as a result of involvement of the sensory portion of the 7th nerve. When the tumour expands beyond the internal auditory canal, the usual signs of a cerebello-pontine angle tumour will be present, including in advanced cases those of increased intracranial pressure.

Cerebrospinal Fluid

Hitselberger and House (1964) have investigated the cerebrospinal fluid protein in 36 patients with acoustic neuroma. Their findings were as follows.

Protein Content in mg/100 ml	Patients	Per cent
0/50	9	25
51/75	8	22
76/100	5	14
101/200	9	25
201/400	3	8
401/700	2	6

They conclude that the smaller tumours are generally associated with relatively minor, if any, changes in the spinal fluid protein content. The finding of a normal fluid protein in the presence of abnormalities revealed by other methods of investigation should not rule out the diagnosis of an acoustic neuroma.

Radiological Diagnosis

Crabtree and House (1964) report on the results of X-ray investigations in 43 cases of proved acoustic neuroma. In 41 there were positive findings. The three views found to be most helpful were the Stenver, the Chamberlain-Towne and the Caldwell, the Stenver being the most helpful. A difference of 1 mm between the diameters of the internal auditory canals on the two sides is suspicious, and, if this difference is accompanied by erosion or difference in shape of the two canals, the findings are strongly suggestive of an acoustic neuroma. Scanlan (1964) reports on the value of positive contrast media in radiography.

SURGICAL TREATMENT OF MÉNIÈRE'S DISEASE

There are now several surgical procedures available for the treatment of Ménière's Disease, some specially indicated in particular cases.

Section of the Vestibular Nerve

This is an old-established procedure aimed at abolishing the vertigo while preserving the hearing. It has no effect upon the tinnitus.

Ultrasonic Irradiation

This technique destroys vestibular function by supplying high frequency sound waves to the horizontal canal. It has the advantage of preserving or even improving hearing in the majority of cases, but some reduction of hearing will occur in one-third. It has the disadvantage of occasionally producing temporary facial paralysis thought to be caused by heat liberated by the applicator.

Endolymphatic Subarachnoid Shunt

This operation has the rational basis of attempting to correct the endolymphatic hydrops which is the cause of Ménière's Disease (House, 1962, 1964, 1965). A shunt is created between the saccus endolymphaticus and the subarachnoid space of the posterior fossa, a silicone rubber tube being inserted to maintain the fistula. The best results from this operation are obtained in patients whose hearing level in the speech frequencies averages less than 50 db with greater loss in the low than in the high frequencies. House's (1965) most recent review of 146 cases operated on by this method, many of which were followed for three or four years, states that the vertigo was relieved in 50 per cent and the tinnitus in 34 per cent. Hearing was improved by 15 db or more in 12 per cent of cases. Further hearing loss occurred in 10 per cent. In some cases operated on, there is a tendency for the recurrence of symptoms owing to closure of the tube by arachnoid adhesions. Long-term follow-up has shown that these recurrences may occur one, two, or even three years after surgery. In such cases there is a tendency for further closure to occur if they are operated on again.

Removal of the Utricle

When hearing is already virtually lost, removal of the utricle by the oval window is a simple and satisfactory method of destroying vestibular function, though cochlear function will be lost at the same time.

References

ASCHAN, G., and STAHLE (1956). *Arch. Otolaryng. Suppl.*, 129.

CARMICHAEL, E. A., DIX, M. R., and HALLPIKE, C. S. (1965). *Brain*, **88**, 51.

CRABTREE, J. A., and HOUSE, W. F. (1964). *Arch. Otolaryngol.*, **80**, 695.

DIX, M. R. (1956). *Brit. med. Bull.*, **12**, 119.

DIX, M. R., and HALLPIKE, C. S. (1952). *Ann. Otol.*, **61**, 987.

FITZGERALD, G., and HALLPIKE, C. S., (1942). *Brain.* **65**, 115

GREEN, D. S. (1963). *J. Speech Dis.*, **28**, 31.

HALLPIKE, C. S. (1955). *Postgrad. med. J.*, **31**, 330.

HALLPIKE, C. S. (1965). *Proc. roy. Soc. Med.*, **58**, 185.

HITSELBERGER, W. E., and HOUSE, W. F. (1964). *Arch. Otolaryngol.*, **80**, 706.

HOUSE, W. F. (1962). *Laryngoscope*, **72**, 713.

HOUSE, W. F. (1964). *Arch. Otolaryngol.*, **79**, 338.

HOUSE, W. F. (1965). *Laryngoscope*, **75**, 1547.

JERGER, J. (1960). *J. Speech Res.*, **3**, 274.

JERGER, J. H., SHEDD, J. L., and HARFORD, E. (1959). *Arch. Otolaryngol.*, **69**, 200.

JOHNSON, E. W., and HOUSE, W. F. (1964). *Arch. Otolaryngol.*, **80**, 667.

PULEC, J. L., and HOUSE, W. F. (1964). *Arch. Otolaryngol.*, **80**, 685.

PULEC, J. L., HOUSE, W. F., and HUGHES, R. L. (1964). *Arch. Otolaryngol.*, **80**, 677.

ROSENBERG, P. E. (1958). Clinical Measurement of Tone Decay read before the American Speech and Hearing Association Convention, 1958.

SCANLAN, R. L. (1964). *Arch. Otolaryngol.*, **80**, 698.

VON BÉKÉSY, G. (1947). *Acta Oto-Laryng.*, **35**, 411.

CHAPTER 4

SOME DISORDERS OF MUSCLE

JOHN N. WALTON

INCREASING world-wide interest in diseases of muscle and of the neuromuscular apparatus within the last 20 years has led to a number of major advances in knowledge. To do full justice to all of these many new developments would require a volume on its own. It is my purpose in this chapter simply to highlight a number of the important new developments of the last few years, rather than to give a comprehensive review of the subject. I propose to consider successively recent advances in knowledge concerning the classification and diagnosis of the various forms of progressive muscular dystrophy and of the myotonic disorders, as well as studies which have assisted in the identification of female carriers of the gene responsible for the most severe form of dystrophy. Next I propose to discuss some of the rare but apparently specific forms of congenital myopathy which have been described in recent years, together with new knowledge concerning benign forms of infantile spinal muscular atrophy. The syndrome of polymyositis will then be reviewed briefly with particular reference to its nosology, diagnosis and management, and I shall then review the various periodic paralysis syndromes and glycogen storage diseases of muscle with brief comments upon other metabolic myopathies. Finally some comments upon new developments in our understanding of myasthenia gravis and myasthenic syndromes will be included.

PROGRESSIVE MUSCULAR DYSTROPHY

It has long been assumed, on the basis of pathological and other evidence, that this disease is primarily one of the muscle cell and the process is at present classified as being degenerative in type as there is no evidence available to indicate its fundamental nature. Many authors have concluded that in all probability the various forms of muscular dystrophy will eventually prove to be due to some specific enzymatic or other biochemical defect within the muscle cell or its membrane. Nevertheless, recent work has suggested that the role of the central and peripheral nervous system in the ætiology of muscular dystrophy may have been too readily discarded. It is well recognized that some degree of intellectual backwardness is common in boys suffering from the severe Duchenne variety of the disease and Rosman and Kakulas (1966) have observed abnormalities on neuropathological examination of the brain in some such cases. Furthermore, the classical experiment of Buller, Eccles and Eccles (1960) which demonstrated by means of cross-innervation that the contraction time of muscle fibres could be modified by transposing their nerve supply and the subsequent observations of Romanul (1966), McPherson (1967) and Dubowitz and Newman (1967) which indicate that the histochemical characteristics of muscle fibres may change completely following such cross-innervation experiments, has plainly indicated that the motor nerve has a profound influence upon the behaviour, both physically and chemically, of the muscle cell. It is nevertheless premature to conclude that abnormalities in the nervous system play a fundamental role in the pathogenesis of muscular dystrophy and most authors would agree that we are still justified in defining this disorder as "genetically-determined primary degenerative myopathy" (Walton, 1960, 1963, 1964a, 1964b, 1965a, 1965b, 1966), but this definition can no longer be regarded as entirely satisfactory as there are a number of other myopathies, including for instance central core disease and nemaline myopathy, which are genetically-determined but which are not normally regarded as being muscular dystrophies.

Classification

Classification of the muscular dystrophies is by no means an academic matter as it is the only safe guide to prognosis and genetic counselling. The traditional clinico-anatomical classification has proved to be unsatisfactory both clinically and genetically since if, for instance, one classifies all cases showing pseudohypertrophy into one group, this is then shown to be heterogeneous with several different forms of inheritance and little clinical uniformity. Important contributions to the problems of classification have been made in recent years by Tyler and Wintrobe (1950), Stevenson (1953), Becker (1953, 1957), Walton and Nattrass (1954), Lamy and de Grouchy (1954), Walton (1955, 1956a), Kloepfer and Talley (1958), Morton and Chung (1959), Chung and Morton (1959), Blyth and Pugh (1959) and Dubowitz (1960). In 1966 I suggested that a satisfactory classification of the muscular dystrophies, based upon clinical and genetic criteria, was as follows:

1. Duchenne-type muscular dystrophy
   Sex-linked recessive variety
   (a) Severe
   (b) Benign
   Autosomal recessive variety
2. Limb-girdle muscular dystrophy
   Autosomal recessive
   Sporadic
3. Facioscapulohumeral muscular dystrophy
   Autosomal dominant
4. Distal muscular dystrophy
5. Ocular myopathy, including oculopharyngeal
6. Congenital muscular dystrophy

This classification, based essentially on the clinical criteria originally proposed by Walton and Nattrass (1954), is still not wholly satisfactory and Becker (1957), as well as others, would prefer one based purely upon genetic grounds. There is justification in Becker's suggestion that the eponymous term "Duchenne" should be reserved for the severe sex-linked recessive cases of early onset and comparatively rapid progression and he suggests that the more benign X-linked type of later onset, which I have included in the group of Duchenne-type dystrophy, may well be a different disease. All authors are agreed concerning the consistent clinical pattern and autosomal dominant inheritance of the facioscapulohumeral form, but the nosological status of the limb-girdle variety is less well defined. It is thus doubtful whether cases of early onset with pelvic girdle weakness which resemble clinically the Duchenne type initially but which may occur in both sexes and run a comparatively benign course should be classified as a benign autosomal recessive subvariety of the Duchenne type, as I have done above, or in the category of so-called limb-girdle muscular dystrophy. Controversy, therefore, is bound to continue and many more detailed family studies will be required in many countries of the world, using rigid clinical and genetic criteria, before a final and definitive answer to the problem can be given. Though the nature of the pathological process causing the muscular weakness and wasting in these cases is similar in character though different in tempo in the various groups, there are other features such as striking differences in the degree to which enzymes such as creatine kinase leak into the serum in the different varieties, which strongly suggest that they may in the end prove to be different diseases from the ætiological standpoint. Nevertheless the classification quoted is, in the present state of knowledge, a reasonably satisfactory guide to prognosis and to genetic counselling.

Clinical Features of the Muscular Dystrophies

These depend upon which muscles are first involved by the disease process and upon the rate of progress of the disease. Weakness in the muscles around the pelvic girdle characteristically gives rise to slowness in walking, inability to run, frequent falling, difficulty in climbing stairs or in rising from the floor, and eventually the patients develop accentuation of the lumbar lordosis and a characteristic waddling gait. Climbing up the legs on rising from the floor (Gowers' sign) is a characteristic feature of the condition but is by no means specific for muscular dystrophy as it occurs in any condition in which pelvic girdle muscles are weakened and thus may be seen in various benign forms of spinal muscular atrophy and in poly-myositis (*vide infra*). Weakness in the shoulder girdle gives an un-usually sloping appearance of the shoulders with a tendency for the scapulæ to rise prominently when the patient attempts to abduct the arms. Many patients utilize trick movements by placing one hand beneath the other elbow in an attempt to lift the hand to the face or head. Facial weakness in its characteristic form, as seen in the facioscapulohumeral variety, causes inability to whistle and to pout the lips or to close the eyes, while distal weakness (seen in the distal variety and in myotonic dystrophy) gives rise to weakness of grip and of fine finger movements and foot-drop. Contractures are a common feature of all forms of muscular dystrophy but are seen particularly in the severe Duchenne type and increase as the disease advances. They may result from weakness developing in a group of muscles whose antagonists remain comparatively powerful (this explains the partial foot-drop with turning in of feet and toes which is seen in advancing cases of the Duchenne type and which typically causes the children to walk on their toes; it results from progressive weakness of the anterior tibial group at a time when the calf muscles remain powerful). Contractures may also be due to postural changes which develop in a patient confined to a wheelchair; in such a situa-tion the biceps and hamstrings show a particular tendency to shorten. One of the most important clinical characteristics of all forms of muscular dystrophy is that muscles are picked out by the disease in a curiously selective manner and this is also one of the most difficult features to explain on any theory of pathogenesis. Though there are certain differences in the pattern of muscular involvement seen in the various subvarieties, it is common in the upper limbs, for instance, to find that the serrati and pectoral muscles are weak and atrophic, as are biceps and brachioradialis, while deltoid and triceps remain relatively powerful. In the lower limbs quadriceps and anterior tibials are particularly weakened and the calf muscles are spared, but in some cases of limb-girdle muscular dystrophy the hamstrings and quadriceps appear to be affected to an equal degree. Such a selective pattern of muscular involvement is very strongly suggestive of muscular dystrophy, but a similar affection of individual muscles with sparing of others may also be seen in some of the more benign varieties of spinal muscular atrophy, though it is rarely as consistent.

The Duchenne Type

Since in over 90 per cent of families this condition is due to a sex-linked recessive gene, the vast majority of the cases occur in males, but the small number of affected females can be accounted for by those rare families in which this variety of the disease is inherited by an autosomal recessive mechanism, as mentioned above. Having made this point, it is important to recognize that over half the afflicted boys suffering from the severe form appear to be isolated cases and in these individuals the disease is presumed to have resulted from genetic mutation occurring perhaps in the cells of one segment of the ovary in either the patient's mother or maternal grandmother. The evidence indicating sex-linked recessive inheritance comes first from the inspection of pedigrees (Walton, 1955), secondly from the fact that several women have been known to have affected children by more than one male (Milhorat and Wolff, 1943; Walton, 1955), thirdly from the finding of families in which there is crossing-over with red-green colour blindness (Philip, Walton and Smith, 1956; Emery, 1966) and fourthly from the fact that two cases of the disease have been reported in patients of female morphology suffering from Turner's syndrome (ovarian agenesis) with an XO chromosome constitution (Walton, 1956a; Ferrier, Bamatter and Klein, 1965). In the severe sex-linked group, which accounts for over 80 per cent of all cases, the disease usually begins in the first three years of life but in about 10 per cent of families showing sex-linked recessive inheritance the condition is more benign and of later onset, beginning usually in the second decade but occasionally as late as the third (Becker, 1957).

In all cases of the Duchenne type the pelvic girdle muscles are first affected clinically but involvement of the shoulder girdles soon follows. Enlargement of the calf muscles and sometimes of quadriceps, deltoids and other muscles as well occurs in about 90 per cent of cases at some stage but later disappears as the disease advances. This enlargement has often been referred to as pseudohypertrophy in view of the fact that muscle biopsy may demonstrate a massive infiltration of fat, but there is good histological evidence now to suggest that in many cases, particularly in the benign sub-variety, this enlargement is due to a true muscular hypertrophy with enlargement of individual muscle fibres. Most patients show slow progressive deterioration so that the majority are unable to walk by the time they are 10 years old, but many patients in the milder sex-linked recessive and autosomal recessive sub-groups continue to walk into early adult life. False or apparent clinical improvement may occur between the ages of 5 and 8 years when the rate of deterioration due to the disease is apparently outstripped by the processes of normal physical development. Once the child is confined to a wheelchair progressive deformity with muscular contractures and skeletal distortion and atrophy occur and death usually results from inanition, respiratory infection or cardiac failure towards the end of the second decade. Some of these children waste progressively but others become excessively obese and no explanation for this discrepancy is forthcoming. Macroglossia is commonly seen and so too is absence of certain incisor teeth (Dubowitz, 1960). The intelligence quotient in these cases is 10 per cent or more lower than in a group of control children of comparable age and sex (Jarvis and Gibson, 1960; Allen and Rodgin, 1960; Dubowitz, 1965; Murphy, Thompson, Corey and Conen, 1965). Marked skeletal atrophy and deformity occur and the shafts of long bones may become pencil-thin and fracture on minimal trauma (Walton and Warrick, 1954). Many patients show clinical evidence of cardiomyopathy with abnormalities in the electrocardiogram (Manning and Cropp, 1958; Levin, Baens and Weinberg, 1959; Skyring and McKusick, 1961; Gilroy, Cahalan, Berman and Newman, 1963); these include prolongation of the P-R interval, slurring of the QRS complex, bundle-branch block, elevation or depression of the ST segment and other changes indicating conduction defects or myocardial degeneration.

Limb-girdle Muscular Dystrophy

This form of the disease occurs equally in the two sexes and usually begins in the second or third decade of life, but occasionally it first appears in middle life. Though genetic evidence plainly indicates that in most families the condition is inherited by an autosomal recessive mechanism and its incidence is therefore considerably increased by consanguinity (Walton, 1955, 1956a), many cases are sporadic and it has been suggested that some may be due to manifestation in the heterozygote (Morton and Chung, 1959; Chung and Morton, 1959). In about half the cases muscle weakness begins in the shoulder girdle muscles and may then remain limited to these for many years before eventually spreading to involve the pelvic girdle. In the other half, by contrast, the pelvic girdle muscles are first involved and as a rule the weakness spreads to the shoulders in about 10 years. Enlargement of calf muscles is not uncommon in these cases. The severity of the disease varies a good deal from case to case and from family to family. Often muscular weakness and wasting are asymmetrical initially and sometimes the disease process appears temporarily to arrest, but in most patients the degree of disability is severe within 20 years of the onset. There is some evidence to suggest that in the patients in whom weakness begins in the upper limbs the disease runs a more benign course than in those in whom the pelvic girdle muscles are first involved. There may be considerable difficulty in distinguishing cases beginning in the pelvic girdle on purely clinical grounds from cases of benign spinal muscular atrophy (vide infra); electromyography is of particular value in making this distinction. Contractures and skeletal deformity occur late in the course of this disease by comparison with the Duchenne type, but progress much more rapidly when the patient is unable to walk. Most sufferers are severely disabled in middle life and many die before the normal age.

Facioscapulohumeral Muscular Dystrophy

This form also occurs equally in the two sexes and can begin at any age from childhood until adult life, though it is usually recognized first in adolescence. Inheritance is by an autosomal dominant mechanism (Tyler and Wintrobe, 1950; Stevenson, 1953; Becker, 1953; Walton, 1955, 1956a; Morton and Chung, 1959) though some families show apparent sex-limitation. Some authors have suggested a possible autosomal recessive mode of inheritance in certain families, but if this does occur it is very uncommon. Facial involvement is apparent at an early stage and is generally accompanied by weakness of shoulder girdle muscles which is often remarkably selective with bilateral winging of the scapulæ and involvement of the pectoral muscles but with sparing of others. Biceps and brachioradialis are often selectively involved and there is difficulty in raising the arms above the head. Muscular hypertrophy or pseudohypertrophy is uncommon in these cases but may be seen in the calves and deltoids. In the lower extremities many such patients show selective involvement of the anterior tibial muscles with bilateral foot-drop and some few, showing unusually rapid progress, demonstrate a particularly severe accentuation of the lumbar lordosis at a comparatively early stage of the disease. The condition which has been referred to as scapuloperoneal muscular dystrophy is probably no more than a variant of this form. In the majority of cases and families the condition is benign, runs a prolonged course with periods of apparent arrest, and muscular contractures and skeletal deformity are late in developing. There are some patients in whom the disease process is apparently abortive and after certain muscles are selectively involved spread of weakness appears to cease spontaneously. Patients tend to show a very characteristic pouting appearance of the lips with a typical transverse smile; most affected individuals survive and remain active until a normal age. Cardiac involvement is rare in this form of muscular dystrophy and in the limb-girdle type and the range of intelligence is normal.

Distal Muscular Dystrophy

This form of the disease is rare in Britain and in the United States, but Welander (1951, 1957, 1966) has reported her experience with over 250 cases of this type. In her experience the condition is inherited as an autosomal dominant character, begins usually between the ages of 40 and 60 and affects both sexes, though it seems to be commoner in men than in women. Weakness begins in the small muscles of the hands and in the anterior tibial muscles and calves, but eventually it spreads proximally, in contradistinction to the weakness observed in peroneal muscular atrophy (Charcot-Marie-Tooth disease) with which this disorder is most often confused. The condition in Sweden is comparatively benign and slowly progressive. Sporadic cases seen in other countries in the world tend to show a rather more rapid course and more severe disability (Barnes, 1932; Milhorat and Wolff, 1943; Walton and Nattrass, 1954). Many workers now believe that the condition which Biemond (1955, 1966) has entitled "myopathia distalis juvenilis hereditaria" is not a myopathy but a variant of peroneal muscular atrophy.

Ocular Myopathy

This disorder usually begins with progressive bilateral ptosis (Hutchinson, 1879; Fuchs, 1890; Kiloh and Nevin, 1951). It used to be generally referred to in the literature as progressive nuclear ophthalmoplegia, but the work of Kiloh and Nevin (1951) and others has demonstrated that the condition is due to a true myopathy of the external ocular muscles even when it occurs in patients also suffering from heredofamilial disease of the nervous system, some of whom also demonstrate pigmentary retinal degeneration (Walsh, 1957; Erdbrink, 1957; Walton, 1964b). Diplopia is rare and in most cases bilateral external ophthalmoplegia develops slowly and progressively over a period of many years. Usually there is also some weakness in the upper facial muscles and often the neck and shoulder girdle muscles are affected to some extent. The facial weakness is particularly severe in the orbicularis oculi but is not as intense as that seen in facioscapulohumeral muscular dystrophy. In 1962 Victor, Hayes and Adams suggested that some such cases demonstrating dysphagia should be classified in a separate group which they entitled "oculopharyngeal muscular dystrophy". Bray, Kaarsoo and Ross (1965) have confirmed this suggestion as they found that in patients with dysphagia the mean age of onset of symptoms was 40 years, but in patients showing ocular myopathy without dysphagia it was 23 years. Barbeau (1965, 1966) has recently shown that many patients with oculopharyngeal muscular dystrophy reported from several centres appear to be descendants of a single French-Canadian family which he has investigated in detail. Plainly ocular myopathy without pharyngeal involvement and the oculopharyngeal variety must be closely related. Genetic information is somewhat confused in that although most families with the oculopharyngeal form show dominant inheritance, many of the purely ocular cases are sporadic, while in other families there has been evidence suggesting sometimes autosomal recessive and sometimes autosomal dominant inheritance (Kiloh and Nevin, 1951).

Congenital Muscular Dystrophy

It was Batten who in 1909 suggested that the syndrome of amyotonia congenita as first described by Oppenheim (1900) might be due to a simple atrophic myopathy of congenital origin. Silvestri (1909) and de Lange (1937) described hypotonic infants with progressive muscular weakness in whom pathological examination suggested that the disease process was one of muscular dystrophy. In 1957 Banker, Victor and Adams described two sibs, one of whom showed widespread muscular weakness and multiple contractures present from birth with a clinical picture of arthrogryposis multiplex congenita; in this case histological examination of the muscle demonstrated a dystrophic process. Short (1963) reported another case with post-mortem findings, and Gubbay, Walton and Pearce (1966) have recently reported detailed clinical and pathological studies of such a case in a child of 4 years. The nosological position of this condition remains unclear. It is plain that there are certain cases in which muscular weakness is present from birth and in which there may or may not be contractures suggesting arthrogryposis and in which histological examination of the muscle reveals undoubted dystrophic change. In some such individuals the disease progresses rapidly and death occurs within the first year of life, but there are some other patients in whom the disease process has seemed virtually non-progressive over a period of several years in that the children, though unable to stand or walk, have not deteriorated. These cases must be distinguished from the various types of benign congenital and relatively non-progressive myopathy to be described below.

Treatment of the Muscular Dystrophies

Regrettably there is no evidence to suggest that any form of drug treatment has any influence upon the course of the disease. Many remedies have been tried in the past and found wanting and none is to be recommended for routine administration, though complications such as respiratory infection may demand appropriate antibiotics. There is, however, good evidence to suggest that physical exercise is of value in delaying the march of the weakness and the onset of contractures and it is advisable to institute a regular programme of exercise which may be started under the supervision of a skilled physiotherapist and subsequently continued at home by the parents who should be given appropriate instructions. Passive stretching of those tendons, such as the tendons of Achilles, which show a tendency to shorten should also be carried out regularly, particularly in the Duchenne type of muscular dystrophy. In certain selected cases the wearing of light spinal supports is helpful in delaying skeletal deformity, and occasionally calipers and night splints are successful in helping affected individuals to walk for longer than they would be able to do without such aids. In general, surgical lengthening of shortened tendons is contra-indicated as the immobilization associated with the surgical procedures often causes deterioration. Not least in importance is the psychological management of these patients, which may demand considerable reserves of patience and understanding on the part of parents, doctors, nurses and social workers. Optimism and encouragement, however unjustifiable in the face of continuing deterioration, are essential.

MYOTONIC DISORDERS

Myotonia is a phenomenon of continued active contraction of the muscle which persists after voluntary innervation ceases; an electrical after-discharge in the electromyogram can be observed to accompany the phenomenon. Three hereditary syndromes, all with autosomal dominant inheritance, have been described, namely myotonia congenita, dystrophia myotonica and paramyotonia congenita. Only in one of these, namely dystrophia myotonica, are dystrophic changes observed within the affected muscles. Transitional cases may be seen suggesting a close relationship between the three disorders and Maas and Paterson (1939, 1950) suggested that these syndromes are merely different manifestations of the same disorder. However, the difference between the course and prognosis of typical cases of dystrophia myotonica on the one hand and of myotonia congenita on the other, and the fact that in the vast majority of families the conditions breed true, suggest that for the present they should be regarded as different diseases. The evidence on this question has been reviewed by Caughey and Myrianthopoulos (1963). Further nosological problems arise over the close relationship between paramyotonia and the periodic paralyses.

Myotonia Congenita

Myotonia congenita (Thomsen, 1876; Nissen, 1923; Thomasen, 1948) usually begins at birth but symptoms may be delayed until the end of the first or even into the second decade. Myotonia is usually generalized, giving painless stiffness which is accentuated by rest and cold and gradually relieved by exercise. It is particularly easy to demonstrate this phenomenon by asking the patient to grip firmly and then to relax, when difficulty in opening the hand will be experienced. The phenomenon can also be demonstrated by percussion of affected muscles and is often well seen in the thenar eminence and tongue; percussion in either situation results in the formation of a dimple in the muscle which only slowly disappears. Diffuse hypertrophy of muscles usually persists throughout life in these cases, though the myotonia tends to improve. Rarely myotonia may increase during exertion (myotonia paradoxa) when it must be distinguished from the cramping stiffness of McArdle's disease. Hypertrophia musculorum vera (Friedreich, 1863; Spiller, 1913) may well be a variant of this condition.

Dystrophia Myotonica

Dystrophia myotonica (myotonia atrophica) was described by Steinert (1909) and Batten and Gibb (1909) and has been reviewed by Thomasen (1948) and Caughey and Myrianthopoulos (1963). It is a diffuse systemic disorder in which myotonia and distal muscular atrophy are accompanied by cataracts, frontal baldness in the male, gonadal atrophy, cardiomyopathy, impaired pulmonary ventilation, mild endocrine anomalies, bone changes, mental defect or dementia and abnormalities of the serum immunoglobulins. The affected families show progressive social decline in successive generations, diminished fertility and an increased infantile mortality rate. The presenting symptom of the condition is usually weakness in the hands, difficulty in walking and frequent falling and myotonia is only rarely obtrusive. Poor vision, loss of weight, impotence or loss of libido, ptosis and increased sweating are common. The condition is usually observed to begin between the ages of 20 and 50 but clinical features of the disorder may be recognized in offspring of affected individuals in the second decade. Recently it has become apparent that the condition may present in infancy and childhood with severe muscular weakness and hypotonia and delay in walking and these children may erroneously be regarded as examples of benign congenital hypotonia unless the existence of myotonic dystrophy in other members of the family is recognized (Vanier, 1960; Dodge, Gamstorp, Byers and Russell, 1965; Pruzanski, 1966).

The facial appearance is characteristic; ptosis and involvement of other external ocular muscles may be seen. Wasting of the masseters, temporal muscles and sternomastoids is almost invariable and in the extremities there is distal weakness and wasting involving mainly forearm muscles, the anterior tibial group and the calves and peronei. Slit-lamp examination reveals cataracts in about 90 per cent of cases. Cardiac involvement is very common and the pulmonary vital capacity and maximum expiratory pressure are often impaired (Kilburn, Eagan, Sieker and Heyman, 1959; Kaufman, 1965); as a result, many patients tolerate barbiturate anæsthesia poorly. Disordered œsophageal contraction can often be demonstrated by contrast radiography or manometry. The testes are usually small and histologically the changes in these organs resemble those of Klinefelter's syndrome though the nuclear sex is male. Irregular menstruation and infertility and prolonged parturition are common in affected females. Pituitary function is usually normal but there may be a selective failure of adrenal androgenic function and occasionally thyroid activity and glucose utilization are impaired (Marshall, 1959; Caughey and Myrianthopoulos, 1963). Hyperostosis of the skull vault, localized or diffuse, and a small sella turcica are frequent radiological findings (Jequier, 1950; Caughey, 1952; Walton and Warrick, 1954). Both mental defect and progressive dementia occur. Rosman and Kakulas (1966) have described neuronal heterotopias in the brain at autopsy in 4 cases and investigation in life may reveal a high incidence of abnormality in the electroencephalogram (Barwick, Osselton and Walton, 1965) or progressive cerebral ventricular enlargement (Refsum, Lounum, Sjaastad and Engeset, 1967). Excessive catabolism of immunoglobulin-G has been demonstrated in these patients by Wochner, Drews, Strober and Waldmann (1966).

Most patients show progressive deterioration and become severely disabled and unable to walk within 15-20 years of the onset. Death from respiratory infection or cardiac failure usually occurs well before the normal age.

Paramyotonia Congenita

This condition, first described by Eulenburg (1886), is characterized by myotonia which is apparent only on exposure to cold, and in addition the patients experience attacks of unexplained generalized muscular weakness similar to those of familial periodic paralysis. The condition is closely related to hyperkalæmic periodic paralysis or adynamia episodica hereditaria (Gamstorp, 1956) (*vide infra*).

The Treatment of Myotonia

In dystrophia myotonica no treatment is known which will influence the progressive muscular wasting and weakness which eventually develops. In paramyotonia the treatment of the attacks of periodic paralysis is similar to that required in patients with familial periodic paralysis of the hyperkalæmic type (*vide infra*). The phenomenon of myotonia may, however, be substantially relieved by means of appropriate drugs. These are particularly valuable in patients with myotonia congenita but are also helpful in some patients with myotonic dystrophy in whom the myotonia is severe. Of drugs used in the past, including quinine, prednisone and procaine amide, the latter is probably the most successful in a dosage of 250–500 mg three or four times daily, depending upon tolerance (Leyburn and Walton, 1959), though the slight risk of agranulocytosis in patients treated with this remedy should be borne in mind. Recently it has been shown (Munsat, 1967) that if anything hydantoin sodium ("Epanutin", "Dilantin") is even more successful in a dosage of 100 mg three times daily.

DIAGNOSTIC METHODS

The value of muscle biopsy in the diagnosis of muscular dystrophy has been recognized since the days of Wilhelm Erb. In recent years, however, the techniques of electromyography and of serum enzyme estimation have added considerable precision to diagnosis.

Electromyography

In neuropathic disorders, spontaneous fibrillation potentials may be recorded from muscle undergoing an active process of denervation, while the pattern of motor unit activity on volition, though reduced from the normal, clearly indicates that the surviving motor unit action potentials are either normal or increased in size and duration. In myopathic disorders, by contrast, spontaneous activity in the form of fibrillation potentials is uncommon, but this type of discharge has been found in some cases of muscular dystrophy though it is more often seen in polymyositis (Walton and Adams, 1958). In patients with myotonia the characteristic type of discharge taking the form of chains of oscillations of high frequency is seen and it is characteristic that these discharges wax and wane in frequency and amplitude and slowly decline and they can be evoked by movement of the exploring needle electrode. Superficially similar spontaneous discharges, often referred to as "pseudomyotonic" in type, are occasionally recorded from various forms of non-myotonic myopathy including polymyositis and various metabolic disorders of muscle, though they are also occasionally seen in non-myotonic dystrophy and in spinal muscular atrophy. It is characteristic of pseudomyotonic discharges that the high frequency discharges remain constant in frequency and amplitude and that they cease abruptly. Volitional activity in the myopathic disorders demonstrates a breakdown of the motor unit action potentials corresponding to patchy degeneration of muscle fibres and as a result there is an increase in short-duration and polyphasic motor unit action potentials (Kugelberg, 1947; Walton, 1952). Buchthal, Rosenfalck and Erminio (1960) have shown that a decrease in the mean action potential voltage and duration together with a reduced motor unit territory and fibre density is seen particularly in the Duchenne type muscular dystrophy, while Buchthal and Pinelli (1953) found that the mean duration of the motor unit action potentials was decreased by up to 60 per cent and the incidence of polyphasic potentials was increased three times in polymyositis. In limb-girdle and facioscapulohumeral muscular dystrophy, however, Buchthal (1962) found that in approximately 50 per cent of cases the mean motor unit action potential duration fell within the normal range. Farmer, Buchthal and Rosenfalck (1959) found the absolute refractory period of voluntary muscle to be reduced in cases of muscular dystrophy. Thus the major value of electromyography is in distinguishing between myopathic disorders on the one hand and neuropathic causes of muscular wasting on the other; it is also valuable in recognizing myotonia, but is of less value in distinguishing between muscular dystrophy on the one hand and other forms of myopathy on the other.

Biochemical Diagnosis

The biochemical abnormalities which have been described in muscular dystrophy and in the other myopathies have been reviewed by Pennington (1965). Excessive creatinuria is observed in many forms of myopathy, as in aminoaciduria in a proportion of cases, but these changes lack specificity. Sibley and Lehninger (1949) first demonstrated that the serum aldolase was raised in patients with progressive muscular dystrophy and subsequently many authors have used the assay of this enzyme in diagnosis. Evans and Baker (1957), Dreyfus, Schapira and Schapira (1958), Thomas, Leyburn and Walton (1960) and many others have found that the activity of this enzyme is raised to about 10 times the normal upper limit in early cases of the Duchenne type muscular dystrophy, while less striking increases are observed in the other more benign varieties. Pearson (1957) showed that similar though less striking increases occurred in the serum activity of the transaminases (aminotrans-ferases) and pointed out that a substantial rise in enzyme activity might occur long before overt clinical signs of the Duchenne type dystrophy appeared, that is in the preclinical phase of the disease. A major advance resulted from the discovery by Ebashi, Toyokura, Momoi and Sugita (1959) that there was a pronounced increase in serum creatine kinase activity in patients with muscular dystrophy. It is now apparent that estimation of this enzyme in the serum is much the most sensitive early diagnostic test for muscular dystrophy of the Duchenne type and that, like the transaminases, this enzyme is greatly raised in the serum in the preclinical stage of the disease. Rises in the activity of this enzyme in the serum are much less striking in other forms of muscular dystrophy and in other muscle diseases and in Table 5 (from Pennington, 1965) I give comparative figures in international units per litre for serum creatine kinase activity obtained in a variety of such disorders. The activity of this enzyme is at its highest in the early stages of all forms of muscle

TABLE 5. SERUM CREATINE KINASE ACTIVITY IN VARIOUS
DISEASES AFFECTING MUSCLE*
(Data from Pearce, Pennington and Walton, 1964)

	No. Examined	No. Elevated	Maximum Level
Muscular dystrophy (Duchenne)	25	25	23,000
Muscular dystrophy (limb-girdle)	6	4	1,650
Muscular dystrophy (facioscapulohumeral)	7	7	301
Dystrophia myotonica	7	5	150
Polymyositis	12	4	1,985
Other myopathies[1]	17	0	—
Neurogenic muscle diseases[2]	14	0	—

Upper limit of normal = 60 I.U. at 37°C.

* From Pennington (1965).

[1] Rheumatoid disease with myopathy (1), carcinomatous myopathy (2), thyrotoxic myopathy (2), rheumatoid disease, steroid treated (2), polymyalgia rheumatica (2), systemic sclerosis (1), dermatomyositis (1), steroid myopathy (6).

[2] Cervical spondylosis (1), polyradiculopathy with muscular wasting (2), multiple sclerosis (1), syringomyelia (1), lumbar spondylosis (1), neuralgic amyotrophy (1), cauda equina compression (1), Dejerine-Sottas syndrome (1), T1 root compression with muscular atrophy (1), motor neurone disease (3), Werdnig-Hoffmann disease (1).

disease and tends to decline as the disease advances. In the Duchenne type dystrophy the activity is probably highest at about the second or third year of life and declines progressively after the age of 10; a similar reduction is seen during the course of limb-girdle and facioscapulohumeral dystrophy, while in polymyositis the activity is highest in acute cases before treatment but a rapid decline occurs following treatment, particularly if it is effective (Rose and Walton, 1966). Another enzyme which is raised in the serum in cases of muscular dystrophy is lactate dehydrogenase, but a more important finding is that abnormalities in the isoenzymes of lactic dehydrogenase have been found on studying muscle biopsy specimens obtained from patients with muscular dystrophy. Patients with this disease often lack LD5, but it now appears that this change, which is also seen in some neurogenic atrophies, is in no sense specific and may simply imply an apparent reversion to the foetal state

(Wieme and Herpol, 1962; Dreyfus, Demos, Schapira and Schapira, 1962; Emery, 1965a; Pearson, 1966).

Histological Diagnosis

I do not propose to review the changes observed in muscle biopsy sections in cases of muscular dystrophy in any detail as these are well-known. The major abnormalities include marked variations in fibre size, fibre splitting, the central migration of sarcolemmal nuclei, patchy atrophy of some fibres and hypertrophy of others, the formation of nuclear chains, areas of necrosis with phagocytosis of necrotic sarcoplasm and basophilia of sarcoplasm with an enlargement of sarcolemmal nuclei showing prominent nucleoli (these changes are construed as being due to abortive regeneration); infiltration with fat cells and connective tissue is also observed. Similar changes may be seen in certain cases of polymyositis (Walton and Adams, 1958; Pearson, 1964) in which disease, however, signs of muscle fibre destruction and repair are usually more striking and widespread and there may be collections of inflammatory cells between the fibres and around blood vessels. It is of some interest that abnormalities are, however, particularly striking in muscle obtained by biopsy from preclinical cases of the Duchenne type (Pearson, 1962; Hudgson, Pearce and Walton, 1967). It is apparent that in this early stage of the disease many muscle fibres are abnormal and profuse abortive regenerative activity is seen, suggesting that the muscle is making a strenuous effort to repair itself from the effects upon it of some pathogenic agent or biochemical deficiency.

Changes observed in biopsy samples obtained from dystrophic patients when studied with the electron microscope have been reviewed recently by Milhorat, Shafiq and Goldstone (1966); as yet no specific ultrastructural abnormality has been discovered in such cases.

X-LINKED DUCHENNE TYPE DYSTROPHY—THE DETECTION OF CARRIERS

There have been considerable advances in recent years in methods of recognizing those female carriers who are likely to pass on the gene responsible for the severe sex-linked recessive variety of the disease to their sons. It is less certain whether these methods are of value in the benign sex-linked families. Since any proven carrier is likely to transmit the disease to half her sons and half her daughters will themselves be carriers, this information is clearly of very considerable importance. Attempts in the past to identify carriers with estimations of creatine and creatinine excretion and of serum aldolase activity (Chung, Morton and Peters, 1960; Schapira, Dreyfus, Schapira and Demos, 1960; Leyburn, Thomson and Walton, 1961; Dreyfus and Schapira, 1962) were somewhat disappointing, as was measurement of limb-to-limb circulation time (Schapira, Dreyfus, Schapira and Demos, 1960). Estimation of the serum creatine kinase has, however, proved to be much more useful (Hughes, 1962; Richterich, Rosin, Aebi and Rossi, 1963; Pearce, Pennington and Walton, 1964; Dreyfus, Schapira, Demos, Rosa and Schapira, 1966) and it now appears that upwards of two-thirds of female carriers may show a rise in serum creatine kinase activity in single samples. Physical exercise, suggested as a possible provocative test for increasing enzyme activity in carriers (Stephens and Lewin, 1965) has not in our hands produced a greater rise in carriers than in control individuals (Hudgson, Gardner-Medwin, Pennington and Walton, 1967). Emery (1965b) has found that he, too, could detect about 65 per cent of carriers of the severe form of the disease using estimation of this enzyme, but this method was successful in detecting only about 20 per cent of carriers of the benign X-linked variety. Van den Bosch (1963) and Barwick (1963) both found minimal electromyographic abnormalities resembling those of muscular dystrophy in some female carriers, but Davey and Woolf (1965) and Caruso and Buchthal (1965) found that they could identify relatively few carriers with this method, though the latter authors observed a consistent reduction in the refractory period of muscle in some such females; unfortunately, however, this method is difficult and time-consuming. Hausmanowa-Petrusewicz et al. (1965) found increased polyphasic potentials and electrocardiographic abnormalities in a considerable number of carriers, and Willison (1965) reported that an electronic spike-counting method of analysis of the electromyogram may prove to be of value in this regard. More recently Gardner-Medwin (1967) has found that the measurement of mean action potential duration in the electromyogram and the measurement of the percentage of polyphasic potentials appear to be more hopeful methods of detecting carriers than was at one time suggested. In his hands this method was successful in detecting several carriers in whom serum creatine kinase activity was consistently normal, and the combination of biochemical and electrophysiological methods increased the carrier detection rate in his series to just over 90 per cent. It is also apparent that muscle biopsy sections obtained from carriers may show significant pathological changes (Dubowitz, 1963; Emery, 1963, 1965c;

Walton, 1964a; Stephens and Lewin, 1965) and Emery (1965a, 1965b) has found a pattern of LDH isoenzymes in such material similar to that observed in established cases of muscular dystrophy. It thus seems that about two-thirds of female carriers of the severe X-linked form of the disease can be detected with serum enzyme estimation alone. Approximately one half of the remainder, or perhaps slightly more, can be identified by means of quantitative electromyography and/or muscle biopsy, but there remain a small number of women known to be definite carriers on genetic grounds in whom the results of these investigations are all normal. Thus positive abnormalities in a putative carrier are of value for genetic counselling, but negative results are less certain and it is still not possible completely to reassure a young woman who presents herself for these tests that if they are all negative there is no chance of her having a dystrophic child.

CONGENITAL HYPOTONIA AND BENIGN CONGENITAL MYOPATHY

It is well recognized that generalized muscular hypotonia in infancy can be due to a variety of causes. In a survey of 111 floppy infants, Paine (1963) found that 48 were suffering from various forms of cerebral palsy, 28 from mental retardation, 3 from cerebral degenerative disease and 1 from brain tumour. There were 4 cases of spinal muscular atrophy and 4 of myopathy, while 18 were found to have benign congenital hypotonia (Walton, 1956b, 1957). While recent work has clearly indicated a remarkable variability in the clinical course of spinal muscular atrophy in infancy and childhood (Byers and Banker, 1961; Dubowitz, 1964) it has recently become apparent that some floppy infants may be suffering from certain apparently specific though benign disorders of muscle which are relatively non-progressive, though there remain a substantial number of hypotonic infants who show gradual improvement and in whom no other diagnostic label than one of benign congenital hypotonia can reasonably be applied since modern methods of investigation fail to demonstrate any cause for the widespread muscular hypotonia which they manifest. I propose now to consider briefly some of the relatively specific forms of myopathy falling into this category which have been described in recent years.

Central Core Disease

In 1956 Shy and Magee described a family of children in which the affected individuals did not walk until about the age of 4 years.

The patients showed profound and widespread muscular hypotonia and muscle biopsy revealed large muscle fibres, most of which showed one or sometimes two central cores which had different staining properties from other fibrils. Further cases have been described by Bethlem and Meyjes (1960) and by Engel, Foster, Hughes, Huxley and Mahler (1961). Dubowitz and Pearse (1960) found the central core to be devoid of oxidative enzymes and of phosphorylase activity and suggested that it was non-functioning. The condition is plainly benign and genetically-determined, being probably the result of an autosomal recessive gene, but as in the several other conditions described below, its pathogenesis remains obscure.

Nemaline Myopathy

In 1963 Shy, Engel, Somers and Wanko described another congenital non-progressive myopathy in which curious collections of rod-shaped bodies were found within the muscle fibres. It is now apparent that in many such cases the clinical diagnosis can be suspected as these patients usually show not only evidence of a diffuse myopathy, but also facial weakness, a high arched palate, prognathism of the lower jaw and skeletal changes resembling those of arachnodactyly, though none of the other stigmata of Marfan's syndrome are present (Ford, 1960; Conen, Murphy and Donohue, 1963; Engel, Wanko and Fenichel, 1964). Examination of muscle from such cases with the electron miscroscope (Price, Gordon, Pearson, Munsat and Blumberg, 1965; Hudgson, Gardner-Medwin, Fulthorpe and Walton, 1967) has shown that the sub-sarcolemmal rods appear to be due to a selective swelling and degeneration of Z-bands with consequent destruction of myofilaments in the adjacent part of the muscle fibre.

Megaconial Myopathy

In children showing a similar clinical presentation to those of central core disease, yet another form of apparently specific pathological change in muscle has been observed by Shy and Gonatas (1964) and has been further described by Shy, Gonatas and Perez (1966). One patient, an 8-year-old white female suffering from a slowly progressive weakness beginning at about the age of 3, showed marked involvement of all shoulder and pelvic girdle muscles. Routine examination of the muscle biopsy with the light microscope did not reveal any significant abnormality, but ultrastructural investigations demonstrated enormously enlarged mitochondria measuring up to 5 mμ in length in the sub-sarcolemmal region as well as throughout the fibre. Some of these mitochondria contained unusual rectangular crystalline-like inclusions of high density.

Subsequently Shy and his colleagues (Shy, 1966) reported another curious mitochondrial abnormality which they have provisionally entitled "pleoconial myopathy". In these cases enormous numbers of rounded mitochondria were seen within muscle fibres. The patients in whom this abnormality was found showed clinical features similar to those described by Poskanzer and Kerr (1961b) in patients with so-called normokalæmic periodic paralysis. The specificity of this mitochondrial change is still in doubt.

Myotubular Myopathy

In a 9-year-old child with a form of Mobius disease characterized by facial diplegia, external ocular palsies, a decrease in muscle mass, moderate symmetrical muscle weakness and poor development of all somatic muscles, Spiro, Shy and Gonatas (1966) found changes which may represent the first example of cellular arrest in the human. The great majority of the muscle fibres contained central nuclei, often lying in chains, and the appearances in the muscle were very similar to those of the so-called myotubes seen in the normal fœtus in the early months of intra-uterine life.

It is as yet too early to be certain that all of these syndromes represent separate specific disorders of muscle, but it is plain that within the entire field of benign congenital myopathy many new and interesting histological abnormalities of the muscle fibre are being demonstrated by histochemical and ultrastructural techniques.

Treatment

No effective drug treatment is known for any of the syndromes of benign hypotonia and benign myopathy described, though physical exercises in moderation and the prevention of contractures by appropriate physiotherapeutic measures and splints where necessary may be helpful.

BENIGN SPINAL MUSCULAR ATROPHY ARISING IN CHILDHOOD AND ADOLESCENCE

Isolated reports of patients with hereditary juvenile spinal muscular atrophy have appeared in the literature for many years and the status of the condition as an independent entity was established by the paper of Kugelberg and Welander (1956). They described 12 patients in 6 families in which the mode of inheritance suggested that the disorder was due to an autosomal recessive gene. The condition began either between the second and fourth year or in adolescence, the course was a long one from 9 to 40 years, and all but 1 of their patients were still alive at the time of writing. The early symptoms, resembling those of muscular dystrophy, were frequent falling, difficulty in rising from the floor, in running and in climbing stairs. Involvement of the arms was noticed later, but in all cases the weakness and wasting of the limb muscles was proximal. Fasciculation was observed in limb muscles in 9 cases and the reflexes were diminished or absent, often with preservation of the ankle jerks, and there were no signs of corticospinal tract disease. Many of these cases had originally been diagnosed on clinical grounds as suffering from muscular dystrophy, but electromyography clearly demonstrated that the disorder was neuropathic and not myopathic in origin and muscle biopsy revealed signs of denervation atrophy. Subsequently the condition was entitled "pseudomyopathic spinal muscular atrophy" because of its close clinical resemblance to muscular dystrophy. A great many isolated cases and families have been described over the last 10 years and the literature has been reviewed recently by Cotton (1965), by Smith and Patel (1965) and by Gardner-Medwin, Hudgson and Walton (1967). The latter authors described 17 patients all of whom suffered from muscular weakness and wasting which was at some stage progressive and in all investigation demonstrated that the condition was caused by a disorder of anterior horn cells. Three of the patients died, but the others were aged between 4 and 43 years at the time of follow-up and in all of them the course of the disease had been very much more benign than that of typical Werdnig-Hoffmann disease or adult motor neurone disease. Eight of the patients were female and 9 male. Nine of the cases were isolated but the other 8 were 4 pairs of affected sibs. In 2 families there was a marked discordance in clinical manifestations between the 2 affected individuals. In each of these families one child had been hypotonic and severely paralyzed from early in life and had died within the first few years, whereas the second individual had shown muscle weakness of much later onset running an extremely benign course. For this and other reasons, the authors concluded that the condition of so-called pseudomyopathic spinal muscular atrophy is not an independent disease entity but is simply a benign variant of infantile spinal muscular atrophy (Werdnig-Hoffmann disease).

The increasing number of these cases now being reported clearly indicates that many have been overlooked in the past and have probably been labelled incorrectly as cases of muscular dystrophy. It is of some interest to note that a modest rise in serum creatine kinase activity has now been reported by many authors in these cases and muscle biopsy samples, as well as demonstrating clear-cut evidence of grouped atrophy due to denervation, not infrequently show changes which may be misconstrued as being myopathic (Gardner-Medwin, Hudgson and Walton, 1967; Hausmanowa-Petrusewicz *et al.*, 1968).

Treatment

No form of drug treatment is of any value in this condition, but graduated physical exercises and the prevention of contractures and skeletal deformity by appropriate physiotherapeutic means are helpful and management must be directed towards increasing the power of those muscles and portions of muscles which retain a nerve supply.

POLYMYOSITIS

The classification and nosological status of polymyositis remains somewhat controversial. This name is usually given to identify a group of cases in which muscular weakness occurs and is sometimes associated with local muscle pain, tenderness and wasting or with evidence of some form of connective tissue disease. Muscle biopsy generally demonstrates areas of muscle fibre necrosis accompanied by interstitial or perivascular cellular infiltrates, or both, though these are not invariable. The term is commonly used to include cases with florid skin change which are more properly called dermatomyositis; it is usually taken to indicate the so-called idiopathic syndrome and excludes disorders such as polymyalgia rheumatica and also acute myositis resulting from infections with micro-organisms and viruses. The relation of the myopathies seen in sarcoidosis, Sjögren's disease and bronchogenic carcinoma to polymyositis is still somewhat obscure (Pearson, 1964), though with the exception of the specific myasthenic-myopathic syndrome which has been observed in patients with lung cancer, it seems probable that most cases of so-called carcinomatous myopathy in reality belong within the syndrome of polymyositis (Rose and Walton, 1966). Shy in 1962 suggested that these disorders should all be referred to as polymyopathies and should be identified according to their ætiology, while Denny-Brown (1960) preferred a pathological classification and suggested that the term polymyositis should be used only when inflammatory changes were seen in muscle biopsy sections; he regarded as separate entities such disorders as necrotizing myopathy and progressive vacuolar myopathy. Walton and Adams (1958) and Barwick and Walton (1963) came to the conclusion that the term polymyositis should be retained, despite objections, since in many cases the ætiology of the condition remains obscure despite full investigation. Furthermore, a response to steroid therapy suggesting a relationship to diseases of the connective tissue group occurs in some patients with a myopathy in whom muscle biopsy findings are very non-specific. There is evidence to suggest that in occasional cases of polymyositis peripheral nerve involvement occurs and these cases may reasonably be referred to as examples of neuromyositis (McEntee and Mancall, 1965; Bekeny, 1965). The recent work of Dawkins (1965) and Kakulas (1966) demonstrating that polymyositis may be induced in rats by the injection of rabbit muscle in Freund's adjuvant, supports the view that this syndrome in the human may well be the result of hypersensitivity or of autoimmune processes, and thus it is possible to suggest that polymyositis in which there is no evidence to suggest that any tissue other than muscle is involved may be an organ-specific autoimmune disease, while in cases showing involvement of skin or joints it may be regarded as being a feature of a non-organ-specific autoimmune disease. The clear-cut relationship between polymyositis and dermatomyositis on the one hand and malignant disease on the other also suggests that the condition may sometimes be the result of a conditioned autoimmune response in patients suffering from cancer. However, attempts to demonstrate anti-muscle antibodies in the serum of patients with polymyositis have to date failed to confirm the presumed autoimmune character of the disease (Stern, Rose and Jacobs, 1967).

The original clinical classification proposed by Walton and Adams (1958), as modified by Rose and Walton (1966), remains reasonably satisfactory for clinical assessment and is given below:

Group I:

Polymyositis
- Acute, with myoglobinuria
- Subacute or chronic—in early adult life
  - in childhood
  - in middle and late life

Group II: Polymyositis with dominant muscular weakness but with some evidence of an associated collagen disease or dermatomyositis with severe muscular disability and with minimal or transient skin changes.

Group III: Polymyositis complicating severe collagen disease, e.g.

rheumatoid arthritis, or dermatomyositis with florid skin changes and minor muscle weakness.

Group IV: Polymyositis complicating malignant disease (including "carcinomatous myopathy" and dermatomyositis occurring in patients with malignant disease).

It must be accepted that some of the cases classified arbitrarily in these groups, and particularly some of those with myoglobinuria, as well as progressive cases of late onset, may be due to metabolic abnormalities unrelated ætiologically to the group of collagen or connective tissue disorders in which most cases of polymyositis rightfully belong.

Detailed analyses of the clinical manifestations of polymyositis have been given by many authors (Eaton, 1954; Garcin, Lapresle, Gruner and Scherrer, 1955; Pearson and Rose, 1960; Barwick and Walton, 1963; Pearson, 1964) and will not be repeated here. It may, however, be said that muscle pain and tenderness occur in approximately 50 per cent of cases, as does dysphagia. Cutaneous manifestations of some kind are seen in about two-thirds of the total but may be unobtrusive, and about one-third are found to have a Raynaud phenomenon. Pain and stiffness in the joints occurs in less than a quarter of the cases. The muscular weakness involves particularly proximal limb muscles and it is characteristic that neck muscle weakness is common, occurring in about two-thirds of cases so that patients have difficulty in holding up the head. Distal muscles are rarely if ever involved alone, and the same applies to facial weakness and involvement of the external ocular muscles, though there are certain cases in which muscular involvement seems generalized. Contractures develop in about a third of all cases. Myasthenic features are occasionally striking and there may be a partial response to edrophonium or neostigmine, but these drugs usually produce only temporary improvement. The deep tendon reflexes may be depressed but are often surprisingly brisk despite the severity of the muscular weakness. Even without treatment the course of the illness is variable. Sometimes the condition runs a fluctuating course with spontaneous exacerbations and remissions. Progressive deterioration with a fatal termination may be seen, while arrest sometimes occurs and in other patients, particularly in middle age, there is slow insidious progression over many years. Spontaneous recovery may occur in childhood (Nattrass, 1954).

In a recent review of 89 cases observed and studied in north-east England, Rose and Walton (1966) found that 14 patients (16 per cent of the whole series) were found to have associated malignant disease. Three laboratory procedures were found to be of diagnostic value, namely serum enzyme estimation, electromyography and muscle biopsy. The serum creatine kinase was found to be substantially raised in acute cases prior to treatment, the electromyogram was abnormal in 89 per cent and muscle biopsy findings were confirmatory in 63 per cent of the cases in which these investigations were performed. Seventy-five patients in their series had received adequate steroid therapy and in the great majority of these the initiation of treatment was followed by subjective and objective clinical improvement accompanied by a progressive reduction in serum enzyme activity. They found that withdrawal of treatment during the first two years after the onset might result in relapse accompanied by a rebound rise in enzyme activity. In some cases prednisone by mouth was ineffective, but ACTH given by injection produced a clinical response. Most patients required treatment for at least 3 years, but despite large doses of prednisone given in the early stage to some patients, side-effects of treatment were few. The outlook was excellent in patients in clinical groups I and II and no deaths occurred in patients under 30 years of age. Over the age of 30 the mortality rate increased in direct proportion to the patients' ages. Most of the deaths in the fourth and fifth decades were due to disseminated lupus erythematosus or progressive systemic sclerosis, and most of those in the sixth and seventh decades were due to associated malignant disease. There seems to be little doubt that longterm treatment with steroid drugs has greatly modified the course and prognosis of this condition.

POLYMYALGIA RHEUMATICA

Polymyalgia rheumatica (Bagratuni, 1953; Gordon, 1960; Todd, 1961) occurs almost always in elderly patients whose principal complaint is one of widespread muscular pain, often with local tenderness, minor constitutional upset and sometimes general malaise. Muscle weakness is not as a rule demonstrable, though pain may be so severe that movement is restricted and as a result patients are often wrongly diagnosed as suffering from polymyositis. It is characteristic that many patients find it impossible, because of pain, to get out of the bath or out of a low chair without help. Muscle biopsy in these cases is usually negative. Some patients go on to develop rheumatoid arthritis and Paulley and Hughes (1960) have suggested that others develop cranial arteritis, but in my experience this is unusual. In every patient the erythrocyte sedimentation rate is substantially raised, but electromyography, serum enzyme studies and muscle biopsy usually give negative findings. The response to steroid therapy is usually immediate and dramatic. The condition seems to belong to the collagen or connective tissue group, but may well prove to be a disorder of intramuscular connective tissue without actual change in muscle fibres.

ENDOCRINE AND METABOLIC MYOPATHIES

Endocrine Myopathies

Disorders of the Thyroid Gland. Chronic thyrotoxic myopathy has been recognized for many years and is well known to respond to treatment of thyrotoxicosis. It is, however, less well known that an association between thyrotoxicosis and periodic paralysis has been observed, particularly among the Japanese. Okinaka, Shizume, Iino, Watanabe, Irie, Noguchi, Kuma, Kuma and Ito (1957) in a study of over 6,000 cases of hyperthyroidism found that 8·9 per cent of the males and 0·4 per cent of the females had had attacks of periodic paralysis of hypokalæmic type. Adequate treatment of the hyperthryoidism resulted in the disappearance of the attacks, or at least in a marked decrease in their number and severity.

In hypothyroidism it has been well known for many years that muscular hypertrophy with slowness of muscular contraction and relaxation and pain on exertion may occur and may be a cause of pseudomyotonia (Crispell and Parson, 1954; Wilson and Walton, 1959). More recently Aström, Kugelberg and Müller (1961) have suggested that myxœdema may occasionally be associated with a girdle myopathy causing mild proximal weakness and wasting similar to that seen in chronic thyrotoxic myopathy; in their patients there was improvement on treatment with thyroxine.

Disorders of the Pituitary and Adrenal Glands. Widespread muscular weakness with some degree of atrophy has been described in hypopituitarism (Walton, 1960) but the nature of the myopathic change in such cases remains to be elucidated (Shy, 1960). General weakness is also seen in some cases of Addison's disease who improve greatly in muscular strength on treatment of the disorder.

In 1959 Müller and Kugelberg described 6 patients with Cushing's syndrome of whom 5 had weakness of the muscles of the pelvic girdle and thighs. Electromyography demonstrated myopathic change in the affected muscles and in the same year Perkoff, Silber, Tyler, Cartwright and Wintrobe (1959) reported cases of muscle weakness and wasting occurring in patients under treatment with steroids. Since that time the naturally-occurring myopathy and the iatrogenic disorder have been frequently reported and it seems that the latter is most often caused by steroids such as triamcinolone which have a fluorine atom in the 9α position (Harman, 1959). Current evidence suggests that the myopathy quickly resolves once the steroid treatment is withdrawn or when the Cushing's disease is effectively treated.

Recently, however, Prineas, Hall and Barwick (1968) have reported the development of proximal muscle weakness and wasting in a series of pigmented patients who had undergone adrenalectomy for the treatment of Cushing's disease. Investigation clearly demonstrated that these patients were suffering from a myopathy and muscle biopsy sections showed a remarkable accumulation of fat within individual muscle fibres. It was concluded that this myopathy was the result of an excessive amount of circulating ACTH.

Metabolic Myopathies

Myopathy in Metabolic Bone Disease. Prineas, Mason and Henson (1965) described two patients with chronic muscular weakness, one of whom had a parathyroid adenoma with osteomalacia and the other was found to be suffering from osteomalacia and idiopathic steatorrhœa. The main clinical features were proximal muscular wasting and weakness, pain and discomfort on movement, with hypotonia and brisk tendon reflexes. They suggested that in these cases a disturbance of vitamin D metabolism could interfere with the excitation-contraction coupling involving the entry of calcium into the muscle fibre during contraction.

Glycogen Storage Disease of Muscle. In 1951 McArdle described the case of a man of 30 who had muscular pain and stiffness which increased during slight exertion. He showed that the blood lactate and pyruvate levels failed to rise after exercise and suggested that the disorder was due to a defect of glucose utilization. In 1959 two additional cases were reported (Schmid and Mahler, 1959; Mommaerts, Illingworth, Pearson, Guillory and Seraydarian, 1959) and one of these also showed myoglobinuria. In both cases muscle glycogen content was increased and myophosphorylase activity was absent. Mellick, Mahler and Hughes (1962) described another case of myophosphorylase deficiency in which there was permanent muscular weakness in the girdle muscles, and Schmid and Hammaker (1961) described three cases in a single family in which the pattern of inheritance suggested an autosomal recessive mechanism; recently Adamson, Salter and Pearce (1967) have also described 3 cases of variable severity in a single family. Engel, Eyerman and

Williams (1963) described 2 patients, one of whom had severe muscular weakness and wasting without cramps developing in late life, while a second, also in middle age, developed cramps after exercise without weakness and wasting and both patients showed a partial defect of muscle phosphorylase activity with a normal total glycogen content in the muscle.

It has become increasingly apparent in recent years that other forms of muscle glycogenosis, though rare, are more common than was at one time realized. In a child of 4 with a diffuse myopathy, Thomson, MacLaurin and Prineas (1963) demonstrated a defect of phosphoglucomutase, and more recently Tarui, Okuno, Ikura, Tanaka, Suda and Nishikawa (1965) have also described a myopathic disorder resembling McArdle's disease which was demonstrated to be the result of phosphofructokinase deficiency. It has been well recognized for many years that the condition now called limit dextrinosis (Illingworth, Cori and Cori, 1956) gives glycogen storage in liver, skeletal muscle and in heart and is due to a deficiency of debranching enzyme (amylo-1,6-glucosidase). This condition, however, like Pompe's disease which gives rise to glycogen storage in the heart, skeletal muscles and central nervous system and which is due to amylo-1,4-glucosidase (acid maltase) deficiency, is usually incompatible with survival beyond the first few years of life. However, it has become apparent quite recently that acid maltase deficiency may be much less grave in its prognosis and several cases are now on record in which the patients presented with an apparently progressive myopathy of girdle muscles in late childhood or in adult life (Zellweger, Brown, McCormick and Tu, 1965; Courtecuisse, Royer, Habib, Monnier and Demos, 1965). We recently have observed 2 such cases, one in a Portuguese undergraduate of 18 and the second in a British housewife aged 44; in both cases a diagnosis of limb-girdle muscular dystrophy had been made on clinical evidence elsewhere, but in each of these patients muscle biopsy demonstrated a remarkable degree of glycogen accumulation within skeletal muscle fibres and detailed biochemical investigation revealed a deficiency in acid maltase (Hudgson, Gardner-Medwin, Worsfold, Pennington and Walton, 1968). It seems more than probable that in the years to come more and more specific myopathic disorders related to individual enzyme defects may well be defined. Unfortunately none of these conditions yet appears to be amenable to any form of effective treatment.

In passing, it should also be mentioned that myopathy resulting from severe and prolonged hypoglycæmia has been described in patients suffering from islet cell adenoma of the pituitary (Mulder, Bastron and Lambert, 1956).

Periodic Paralysis and its Variants. The classical hypokalæmic variety of periodic paralysis has been well recognized for many years and recently has been reviewed by McArdle (1964). This condition gives rise to attacks of flaccid weakness of the voluntary muscles but those of speech, swallowing and respiration are usually spared. Attacks most often begin in the second decade and are most frequent in early adult life. Commonly they last for several hours and often start early in the morning on waking, after a period of rest following exertion or after a heavy carbohydrate meal. During attacks the plasma potassium level is usually found to be low (less than 3 mEq/l.); there is positive balance of potassium and some or all of the retained potassium seems to pass into the muscle cell (Grob, Johns and Liljestrand, 1957; Zierler and Andres, 1957). Shy, Wanko, Rowley and Engel (1961) have shown that the resting membrane potential is normal during an attack of paralysis, and these authors and Pearce (1964) have demonstrated that electron microscopy of muscle biopsy specimens taken during an attack show vacuoles resulting from dilatation of the sarcoplasmic reticulum. Conn and Streeten (1960) suggested that this form of periodic paralysis might be due to intermittent aldosteronism as it is well recognized that patients with primary aldosteronism due to tumours of the adrenal (Conn, 1955) do have attacks of muscular weakness. However, aldosteronism can be distinguished from periodic paralysis by the associated hypertension, alkalosis and hypernatræmia and by the persistence of the hypokalæmia between the attacks; furthermore, in familial periodic paralysis increased aldosterone excretion is not usually found. Administration of potassium chloride is the treatment of choice for attacks of the hypokalæmic type but rarely seems to shorten the episodes of weakness. Spironolactone and other aldosterone antagonists have been found, however, to reduce greatly the frequency and severity of the attacks (Poskanzer and Kerr, 1961a). Occasionally in these cases muscular weakness is curiously localized to one or more muscle groups and sometimes after frequent episodes of weakness permanent atrophy of muscles develops, but on the whole the patients tend to improve spontaneously as they grow older.

In 1951 Tyler, Stephens, Gunn and Perkoff described a group of cases in which the serum potassium level did not fall during the attacks and the patients were made worse by potassium chloride. Helweg-Larsen, Hauge and Sagild (1955) described a similar condition and Gamstorp (1956) described two families containing such cases and entitled the condition adynamia episodica hereditaria (hyperkalæmic periodic paralysis is probably a more satisfactory title (Klein, Egan and Usher, 1960)). This condition is closely related to paramyotonia for some of the patients show definite myotonia (Drager, Hammill and Shy, 1958; Van der Meulen, Gilbert and Kane, 1961) though in others the myotonia seems curiously limited to the muscles around the eye and can be evoked by placing ice-bags on the eyelids, a manœuvre which tends to give a remarkable degree of lid-lag. Van't Hoff (1962) has referred to such cases as examples of myotonic periodic paralysis. In affected individuals the attacks are usually much shorter in duration than in the hypokalæmic variety, lasting on an average 30–40 minutes, and they may be precipitated immediately by exercise. Commonly there is a rise in the serum potassium level, though some patients have severe weakness when the level is no higher than 4 mEq/l., whereas in normal people a level of 8 mEq/l. is needed as a rule before weakness develops. Abbott, Creutzfeldt, Fowler and Pearson (1962) have shown that the muscle fibre membrane potential is lowered during the attacks in such cases. The attacks may be cut short by the intravenous administration of calcium gluconate, while acetazolamide, hydrochlorothiazide and dichlorphenamide have all been used successfully for prophylaxis.

The third type of periodic paralysis, entitled provisionally the so-called sodium-responsive normokalæmic variety (Poskanzer and Kerr, 1961b) is probably a variant of the hyperkalæmic type, except for the fact that in these cases the attacks have been seen occasionally to last for days or weeks and have often developed at night. Nevertheless in these patients paralysis is always increased by the administration of potassium and improved by large doses of sodium chloride. It is in cases of this type that Shy and his colleagues (Shy, 1966) have described the appearance of very much increased numbers of mitochondria in muscle biopsy sections examined with the electron microscope and have referred to this change as pleoconial myopathy. Poskanzer and Kerr (1961b) found that acetazolamide combined with 9-α-fluorohydrocortisone, 0·1 mg daily, prevented the attacks.

This recent work has clearly indicated that careful investigation of every case of periodic paralysis is necessary in order to establish the nature of the patient's illness. Attempts to demonstrate a primary enzyme defect or a specific disorder of carbohydrate metabolism in such cases have so far been unsuccessful, but empirical treatment, both given prophylactically or in order to cut short the attacks, has proved to be successful once the character of the patient's attacks has been carefully defined by investigation.

NEW LIGHT ON MYASTHENIA GRAVIS

Classification

As Simpson stated in 1964, many people have doubted whether myasthenia gravis is a disease entity. The symptom of myasthenia is characterized by the development of an abnormal degree of weakness in voluntary muscles following repetitive contraction or prolonged tension with a marked tendency for motor power to recover after a period of inactivity or lessened tension. This type of fatiguability can be observed in muscles affected by polymyositis (Walton and Adams, 1958), systemic lupus erythematosus, dermatomyositis and one type of carcinomatous neuropathy (Anderson, Churchill-Davidson and Richardson, 1953; Lambert, Eaton and Rooke, 1956) and even in some cases of benign congenital myopathy (Walton, Geschwind and Simpson, 1956; Rowland and Eskenazi, 1956). However, a therapeutic response to anticholinesterase drugs is necessary for the definition of true myasthenia gravis, and although some response may be found in the symptomatic myasthenias it is rarely dramatic and often fails within a few weeks. There are, for instance, striking clinical differences between myasthenia gravis *per se* and the carcinomatous myasthenic-myopathic syndrome seen in cases of lung carcinoma, while in the latter condition improvement in muscle power on treatment with guanidine is much more striking than when neostigmine is given (McQuillen and Johns, 1967). Simpson (1964) therefore suggests that despite the occurrence of myasthenia in the broadest sense in other diseases, myasthenia gravis is a clearly recognizable disease entity in which the response to anticholinesterase drugs is dramatic and sustained and it is also a condition with an individual natural history and pathology.

Incidence and Natural History

The clinical picture of myasthenia gravis is well-known and will not be detailed here, but it is important to note that while in many cases the bulbar muscles are particularly involved, in others muscular weakness is widespread but in some cases (Grob, 1953; Ferguson, Hutchinson and Liversedge, 1955) the disease appears to remain limited to the external ocular muscles and never spreads to those of the bulb or limbs. Neonatal myasthenia is seen in about one in seven of the children born to myasthenic mothers (Osserman, 1958) but in those who survive it usually recovers in between a week and 3 months and does not recur.

In general, myasthenia occurs in all races and affects both sexes, but is twice as common in women as in men. It usually develops in early adult life but may begin for the first time in the elderly. Long-lasting remissions are infrequent and most occur within the first 5 years of the disease process (Schwab and Leland, 1953; Simpson, 1964). Most deaths occur within this period and death from the disease is rare after it has been in existence for 10 years, since in many cases the condition appears to be burnt out at this stage. It is not commonly recognized that muscle wasting may occur in long-standing cases and that this is uninfluenced by adequate treatment with anticholinesterase drugs; this wasting with irreversible weakness is most common in the external ocular muscles and in certain limb muscles, particularly the triceps brachii.

Diagnosis

The diagnosis of myasthenia depends not only upon the character-istic clinical picture and upon the fatiguability which may be demon-strated by electrical tests, but also upon the clinical response to an injection of neostigmine (Rowland, 1955) or preferably the short-acting edrophonium hydrochloride (Osserman and Kaplan, 1953); this latter drug, which is given in a dosage of 10 mg intravenously, has now more or less supplanted neostigmine for diagnostic purposes. Provocative tests designed to increase myasthenia, utilizing such drugs as d-tubocurarine and quinine, are dangerous and are generally to be condemned. Churchill-Davidson and Richardson (1952) showed that myasthenic patients are abnormally resistant to the action of certain depolarizing neuromuscular blocking agents such as decamethonium. Tolerance is particularly marked in clinically unaffected muscles. However, depolarization block, if it occurs at all, is brief and soon changes to a longer competitive (curare-like) type of block. This dual response in the child or adult is character-istic of myasthenia gravis, but it is interesting to note that the response obtained in normal neonates is similar (Churchill-Davidson and Wise, 1963).

Ætiology

Simpson (1960, 1964, 1965) has drawn attention to the inter-relationship between myasthenia gravis and a variety of other diseases. An association with thyroid disease has been well known for some years, but he also found that a number of myasthenic patients under his care suffered from disorders such as diabetes, rheumatoid arthritis, systemic lupus erythematosus and sarcoidosis. He therefore suggested in 1960 that myasthenia may well be an autoimmune disorder and that the thymus might produce an antibody against muscle end-plate protein. In 1960 for the first time Strauss, Seegal, Hsu, Burkholder, Nastuk and Osserman demonstrated a muscle-binding globulin in mysasthenic serum and more recently White and Marshall (1962), Oosterhuis, Van der Geld, Feltkamp and Peetoom (1964), Strauss, Smith, Cage, Van der Geld, McFarlin and Barlow (1966) and Van der Geld and Strauss (1966) have confirmed that antimuscle antibodies are present in a high proportion of cases and may be most clearly demonstrated by a fluorescent antibody technique. However, such antibodies were also present in some patients with thymomas who did not have myasthenia. Marshall and White (1961) showed that direct injection of bacterial antigen into the guinea-pig thymus produced a histological reaction similar to that seen in myasthenia, while recently Goldstein and Whittingham (1966) found that 6 of 24 guinea-pigs immunized with either thymus or muscle in complete Freund's adjuvant developed a myasthenic neuromuscular block on electromyographic testing. Thymectomy in 19 animals prevented the development of this block after immunization with thymus or muscle. Histologically the thymus showed changes which could be interpreted as being those of an experimental autoimmune thymitis. The authors concluded that in human myasthenia gravis an autoimmune reaction in the thymus may well liberate a humoral substance which causes the characteristic myasthenic neuromuscular block. Simpson (1966) therefore suggested that myasthenia might be due to an antigen-antibody reaction involving end-plate protein. Recently, however, Housley and Oppenheim (1967) have investigated 3 thymectomized and 3 non-thymectomized patients for possible depression of immunological competence; they studied the response of peripheral blood lymphocytes to homogenates of muscle and of thymus but their results were essentially negative. Desmedt (1957) suggested that the lesion is presynaptic as the disorder of function in myasthenia is closely simulated by the administration of hemicholinium, which impairs acetylcholine synthesis. On the other hand, Dählback, Elmqvist, Johns, Radner and Thesleff (1961), who inserted intracellular electrodes into isolated intercostal muscles removed from myasthenic and control patients, demonstrated a disturbance of transmitter formation or release and also showed that the chemical sensitivity of the post-junctional membrane to acetylcholine was normal. This led them to conclude that the amount of acetylcholine being produced at the motor end-plate was abnormally low in these cases. It is, of course, possible that some kind of autoimmune response may prevent the proper release or formation of this substance. Nevertheless, despite much recent and important work, the exact role of autoimmune mechanisms in myasthenia remains unclear. The presence of morphological abnormalities in terminal nerve endings in myasthenic muscle, as described by Coërs and Desmedt (1959), Bickerstaff and Woolf (1960) and Mac-Dermot (1960) is as yet unexplained but may well be a secondary phenomenon.

Treatment

The standard treatment for myasthenia gravis is still the administration of neostigmine or the closely related drug pyridostigmine. The newer remedy, mytelase, has not proved to be superior to this form of traditional treatment (Osserman, 1958; Simpson, 1965). The differential diagnosis between increasing myasthenic weakness on the one hand and cholinergic weakness on the other can be a matter of considerable difficulty. The most useful single test is to give an intravenous injection of edrophonium; if this increases muscle power, then the weakness is likely to be myasthenic and more treatment is required, while if weakness increases after the injection this suggests that it is cholinergic and that treatment must be reduced. Any sign of impending respiratory insufficiency may be an indication for withdrawal of all drugs and for assisted respiration with positive pressure apparatus and tracheotomy. Unfortunately many patients show a differential response on the part of different muscles to various drugs, depending presumably upon the extent to which the individual muscles are involved by the disease process. In several patients whom I have had under my care a dose of neostigmine or pyridostigmine sufficient to improve power in the limb muscles was sufficient to cause cholinergic paralysis of the diaphragm or bulbar muscles.

The place of thymectomy is still in some doubt. Eaton and Clagett (1950) found no significant improvement in their cases, but Keynes (1946, 1954) pointed out that in the Mayo Clinic series (Eaton and Clagett, 1950) the patients with thymic tumours were not separated from the remainder. Simpson (1958, 1960) reviewed the problem in detail and has pointed out that thymectomy benefits both sexes but that the extent of improvement is greatest for women, who would otherwise have a worse prognosis than men. Benefit following the operation may occur at any time, but the results are best in a young woman with a short history suffering from severe myasthenia.

However, any patient who is deteriorating despite optimum medical treatment has nothing to lose and may improve. The prognosis for life is always worse if a thymoma is present and in these cases radiotherapy is generally recommended prior to operation; nevertheless, even after thymectomy, 2 out of 3 patients suffering from thymomas die within 5 years.

CONCLUSIONS

It has been possible to do little more in this chapter than to draw attention to a number of important advances which have occurred in our understanding of muscle disease within the last 10–15 years, but new developments are occurring at such a rate that without question many recent concepts and classifications will have to be discarded or modified within the next decade. The continuing application of modern methods of genetic, biochemical, pathological, cytological and electrophysiological research will undoubtedly continue to increase our understanding of the behaviour of the neuromuscular apparatus in health and disease.

References

ABBOTT, B. C., CREUTZFELDT, O. D., FOWLER, B., and PEARSON, C. M. (1962). *Fed. Proc.*, **21**, 318.

ADAMSON, D., SALTER, R. H., and PEARCE, G. W. (1967). *Quart. J. Med.*, **36**, 565.

ALLEN, J. E., and RODGIN, D. W. (1960). *Amer. J. Dis. Child.*, **100**, 208.

ANDERSON, H. J., CHURCHILL-DAVIDSON, H. C., and RICHARDSON, A. T. (1953). *Lancet*, **2**, 1291.

ASTRÖM, K. E., KUGELBERG, E., and MÜLLER, R. (1961). *Arch. Neurol. (Chic.)*, **5**, 472.

BAGRATUNI, L. (1953). *Ann. rheum. Dis.*, **12**, 98.

BANKER, B. Q., VICTOR, M., and ADAMS, R. D. (1957). *Brain*, **80**, 319.

BARBEAU, A. (1965). *Proc. 8th int. Congr. Neurol.*, p. 257.

BARBEAU, A. (1966). In *Symposium über progressive Muskeldystrophie*, ed. E. Kuhn. Berlin, Heidelberg, New York, Springer-Verlag.

BARNES, S. (1932). *Brain*, **55**, 1.

BARWICK, D. D. (1963). In *Research in Muscular Dystrophy*, p. 10. London, Pitman.

BARWICK, D. D., OSSELTON, J. W., and WALTON, J. N. (1965). *J. Neurol. Neurosurg. Psychiat.*, **28**, 109.

BARWICK, D. D., and WALTON, J. N. (1963). *Amer. J. Med.*, **35**, 646.

BATTEN, F. E. (1909). *Quart. J. Med.*, **3**, 313.

BATTEN, F. E., and GIBB, H. P. (1909). *Brain*, **32**, 187.

BECKER, P. E. (1953). *Dystrophia Musculorum Progressiva*. Stuttgart, Thieme.

BECKER, P. E. (1957). *Acta genet. (Basel)*, **7**, 303.

BEKENY, G. (1965). *Proc. 8th int. Congr. Neurol.*, p. 581.

BETHLEM, J., and MEYJES, F. E. P. (1960). *Psychiat. Neurol. Neurochir. (Amst.)*, **63**, 246.

BICKERSTAFF, E. R., and WOOLF, A. L. (1960). *Brain*, **83**, 10.

BIEMOND, A. (1955). *Acta psychiat. neurol. scand.*, **30**, 25.

BIEMOND, A. (1966). In *Symposium über progressive Muskeldystrophie*, ed. E. Kuhn. Berlin, Heidelberg, New York, Springer-Verlag.

BLYTH, H., and PUGH, R. J. (1959). *Ann. hum. Genet.*, **23**, 127.

BRAY, G. M., KAARSOO, M., and ROSS, R. T. (1965). *Neurology (Minneapolis)*, **15**, 678.

BUCHTHAL, F. (1962). *Wld. Neurol.*, **3**, 16.

BUCHTHAL, F., and PINELLI. P., (1953). *Neurology (Minneapolis)*, **3**, 424.

BUCHTHAL, F., ROSENFALCK, P., and ERMINIO, F. (1960). *Neurology (Minneapolis)*, **10**, 398.

BULLER, A. J., ECCLES, J. C., and ECCLES, R. M. (1960). *J. Physiol. (Lond.)*, **150**, 399.

BYERS, R. K., and BANKER, B. Q. (1961). *Arch. Neurol. (Chic.)*, **5**, 140.

CARUSO, G., and BUCHTHAL, F. (1965). *Brain*, **88**, 29.

CAUGHEY, J. E. (1952). *J. Bone Jt. Surg.*, **34B**, 343.

CAUGHEY, J. E., and MYRIANTHOPOULOS, N. C. (1963). *Dystrophia Myotonica and Related Disorders*. Springfield, Ill., Thomas.

CHUNG, C. S., and MORTON, N. E. (1959). *Amer. J. hum. Genet.*, **11**, 339.

CHUNG, C. S., MORTON, N. E., and PETERS, H. A. (1960). *Amer. J. hum. Genet.*, **12**, 52.

CHURCHILL-DAVIDSON, H. C., and RICHARDSON, A. T. (1952). *J. Neurol. Neurosurg., Psychiat.*, **15**, 129.

CHURCHILL-DAVIDSON, H. C., and WISE, R. P. (1963). *Anesthesiology*, **24**, 271.

COËRS, C., and DESMEDT, J. E. (1959). *Acta neurol. belg.*, **59**, 539.

CONEN, P. E., MURPHY, E. G., and DONOHUE, W. L. (1963). *Canad. med. Ass. J.*, **89**, 983.

CONN, J. W. (1955). *J. Lab. clin. Med.*, **45**, 661.

CONN, J. W., and STREETEN, D. H. P. (1960). In *The Metabolic Basis of Inherited Disease*, ed. J. B. Stanbury, J. B. Wyngaarden and D. S. Fredrickson, p. 867. New York, McGraw-Hill.

COTTON, J. B. (1965). *Lyon méd.*, **213**, 1295.

COURTECUISSE, V., ROYER, P., HABIB, R., MONNIER, C., and DEMOS, J. (1965). *Arch. franc. Pédiat.*, **22**, 1153.

CRISPELL, K. R., and PARSON, W. (1954). *Trans. Amer. Goiter Ass.*, 399.

DÄHLBACK, O., ELMQVIST, D., JOHNS, T. R., RADNER, S., and THESLEFF, S. (1961). *J. Physiol. (Lond.)*, **156**, 336.

DAVEY, M. R., and WOOLF, A. L. (1965). *Proc. 6th int. Congr. EEG clin. Neurophysiol.*, p. 653.

DAWKINS, R. L. (1965). *J. Path. Bact.*, **90**, 619.

DE LANGE, C. (1937). *Acta pædiat.*, **20**, Suppl. III.

DENNY-BROWN, D. (1960). *Trans. Coll. Phycns. Philad.*, **28**, 14.

DESMEDT, J. E. (1957). *Rev. neurol.*, **96**, 505.

DODGE, P. R., GAMSTORP, I., BYERS, R. K., and RUSSELL, P. (1965). *Pediatrics*, **35**, 3.

DRAGER, G. A., HAMMILL, J. F., and SHY, G. M. (1958). *Arch. Neurol. (Chic.)*, **80**, 1.

DREYFUS, J. C., DEMOS, J., SCHAPIRA F. and SCHAPIRA, G. (1962). *C.R. Acad. Sci., (Paris)*, **254**, 4384.

DREYFUS, J. C., SCHAPIRA, F., DEMOS, J., ROSA, R., and SCHAPIRA, G. (1966). *Ann. N.Y. Acad. Sci.*, **138**, 304.

DREYFUS, J. C., and SCHAPIRA, G. (1962). *Klin. Wschr.*, **40**, 373.

DREYFUS, J. C., SCHAPIRA, G., and SCHAPIRA, F. (1958). *Ann. N.Y. Acad. Sci.*, **75**, 235.

DUBOWITZ, V. (1960). *Brain*, **83**, 432.

DUBOWITZ, V. (1963). *J. Neurol. Neurosurg. Psychiat.*, **26**, 322.

DUBOWITZ, V. (1964). *Brain*, **87**, 707.

DUBOWITZ, V. (1965) *Arch, Dis. Childh.*, **40**, 296.

DUBOWITZ, V., and NEWMAN, D. L. (1967). *Nature*, **214**, 840.

DUBOWITZ, V., and PEARSE, A. G. E. (1960). *Lancet*, **2**, 23.

EATON, L. M. (1954). *Neurology (Minneapolis)*, **4**, 245.

EATON, L. M., and CLAGETT, O. T. (1950). *J. Amer. med. Ass.*, **142**, 963.

EBASHI, S., TOYOKURA, Y., MOMOI, H., and SUGITA, H. (1959). *J. Biochem. (Tokyo)*, **46**, 103.

EMERY, A. E. H. (1963). *Lancet*, **1**, 1126.

EMERY, A. E. H. (1965a). In *Research in Muscular Dystrophy*, 2nd series, p. 90. London, Pitman.

EMERY, A. E. H. (1965b). *J. Genet. hum.*, **14**, 318.

EMERY, A. E. H. (1965c). *J. med. Genet.*, **2**, 1.

EMERY, A. E. H. (1966). *J. med. Genet.*, **3**, 92.

ENGEL, W. K., EYERMAN, E. L., and WILLIAMS, H. E. (1963). *New Engl. J. Med.*, **268**, 135.

ENGEL, W. K., FOSTER, J. B., HUGHES, B. P., HUXLEY, H. E., and MAHLER, R. (1961). *Brain*, **84**, 167.

ENGEL, W. K., WANKO, T., and FENICHEL, G. M. (1964). *Arch. Neurol (Chic.)*, **11**, 22.

ERDBRINK, W. L. (1957). *Arch. Ophthal.*, **57**, 335.

EULENBURG, A. (1886). *Neurol. Zbl.*, **5**, 265.

EVANS, J. H., and BAKER, R. W. R. (1957). *Brain*, **80**, 557.

FARMER, T. W., BUCHTHAL, F., and ROSENFALCK, P. (1959). *Neurology (Minneapolis)*, **9**, 747.

FERGUSON, F. R., HUTCHINSON, E. C., and LIVERSEDGE, L. A. (1955). *Lancet*, **2**, 636.

FERRIER, R., BAMATTER, F., and KLEIN, D. (1965). *J. med. Genet.*, **2**, 38.

FORD, F. R. (1960). *Diseases of the Nervous System in Infancy, Childhood and Adolescence*, 4th edition. Springfield, Ill, Thomas.

FRIEDREICH, N. (1863). *Arch. path. Anat.*, **28**, 474.

FUCHS, E. (1890). *Arch. Ophthal.*, **36**, 234.

GAMSTORP, I. (1956). *Acta pædiat. (Uppsala)*, Suppl. 108.

GARCIN, R. LAPRESLE J., GRUNER, J., and SCHERRER, J. (1955). *Rev. neurol.*, **92**, 465.

GARDNER-MEDWIN, D. (1968). *J. Neurol. Neurosurg. Psychiat.*, in the press.

GARDNER-MEDWIN, D., HUDGSON, P., and WALTON, J. N. (1967). *J. Neurol. Sci.*, **5**, 121.

GILROY, J., CAHALAN, J. L., BERMAN, R., and NEWMAN, M. (1963). *Circulation*, **27**, 484.

GOLDSTEIN, G., and WHITTINGHAM, S. (1966). *Lancet*, **2**, 315.

GORDON, I. (1960). *Quart. J. Med.*, **29**, 473.

GROB, D. (1953). *J. Amer. med. Ass.*, **153**, 529.

GROB, D., JOHNS, R. J., and LILJESTRAND, A. (1957). *Amer. J. Med.*, **23**, 356.

GUBBAY, S. S., WALTON, J. N., and PEARCE, G. W. (1966). *J. Neurol. Neurosurg. Psychiat.*, **29**, 500.

HARMAN, J. B. (1959). *Lancet*, **1**, 887.

HAUSMANOWA-PETRUSEWICZ, I., ASKANAS, W., BADURSKA, B., EMERYK, B., FIDZIANSKA, A., GARBALINSKA, W., HETNARSKA, L., JEDRZEJOWSKA, H., KAMIENIECKA, Z., NIEBROJDOBOSZ, I., PROT, J., and SAWICKA, E. (1968). *J. Neurol. Sci.*, in the press.

HAUSMANOWA-PETRUSEWICZ, I., PROT, J., NIEBROJ-DOBOSZ, I., EMERYK, B., WASOWICZ, B., SLUCKA, C., HETNARSKA, L., BANDARZEWSKA, B., and PUCEK, Z. (1965). *Proc. 8th int. Congr. Neurol.*, p. 635.

HELWEG-LARSEN, H. F., HAUGE, M., and SAGILD, U. (1955). *Acta genet. (Basel)*, **5**, 263.

HOUSLEY, J., and OPPENHEIM, J. J. (1967). *Brit. med. J.*, **1**, 679.

HUDGSON, P., GARDNER-MEDWIN, D., FULTHORPE J. J., and WALTON, J. N. (1967). *Neurology (Minneapolis)*, **17**, 1125.

HUDGSON, P., GARDNER-MEDWIN, D., PENNINGTON, R. J. T., and WALTON, J. N. (1967). *J. Neurol. Neurosurg. Psychiat.*, **30**, 416.

HUDGSON, P., GARDNER-MEDWIN, D., WORSFOLD, M., PENNINGTON, R. J. T., and WALTON, J. N. (1968). *Brain*, in the press.

HUDGSON, P., PEARCE, G. W., and WALTON, J. N. (1967). *Brain*, **90**, 565.

HUGHES, B. P. (1962). *Brit. med. J.*, **2**, 963.

HUTCHINSON, J. (1879). *Med.-chir. Trans.*, **62**, 307.

ILLINGWORTH, B., CORI, G. T., and CORI, C. F. (1956). *J. biol. Chem.*, **218**, 123.

JARVIS, J. M., and GIBSON, J. (1960). Personal communication.

JEQUIER, M. (1950). *Schweiz. med. Wschr.*, **80**, 593.

KAKULAS, B. A. (1966). *J. Neuropath. exp. Neurol.*, **25**, 148.

KAUFMAN, L. (1965). In *Research in Muscular Dystrophy*, 2nd series. London, Pitman.

KEYNES, G. (1946). *Brit. J. Surg.*, **33**, 201.

KEYNES, G. (1954). *Lancet*, **1**, 1197.

KILBURN, K. H., EAGAN, J. T., SIEKER, H. O., and HEYMAN, A. (1959). *New Engl. J. Med.*, **261**, 1089.

KILOH, L. G., and NEVIN, S. (1951). *Brain*, **74**, 115.

KLEIN, R., EGAN, T., and USHER, P. (1960). *Metabolism*, **9**, 1005.

KLOEPFER, H. W., and TALLEY, C. (1958). *Ann. hum. Genet.*, **22**, 138.

KUGELBERG, E. (1947). *J. Neurol. Neurosurg. Psychiat.*, **10**, 122.

KUGELBERG, E., and WELANDER, L. (1956). *Arch. Neurol. Psychiat. (Chic.)*, **75**, 500.

LAMBERT, E. H., EATON, L. M., and ROOKE, E. D. (1956). *Amer. J. Physiol.*, **187**, 612.

LAMY, M., and DE GROUCHY, J. (1954). *J. Genet. hum.*, **3**, 219.

LEVIN, S., BAENS, G. S., and WEINBERG, T. (1959). *J. Pediat.*, **55**, 460.

LEYBURN, P., and WALTON, J. N. (1959). *Brain*, **82**, 81.

LEYBURN, P., THOMSON, W. H. S., and WALTON, J. N. (1961). *Ann. hum. Genet.*, **25**, 41.

MAAS, O., and PATERSON, A. S. (1939). *Brain*, **62**, 198.

MAAS, O., and PATERSON, A. S. (1950). *Brain*, **73**, 318.

MANNING, G. W., and CROPP, G. J. (1958). *Brit. Heart. J.*, **20**, 416.

MARSHALL, A. H. E., and WHITE, R. G. (1961). *Lancet*, **1**, 1030.

MARSHALL, J. (1959). *Brain*, **82**, 221.

MCARDLE, B. (1951). *Clin. Sci.*, **10**, 13.

MCARDLE, B. (1964). Chapter 15, *Disorders of Voluntary Muscle*, ed. J. N. Walton. London, Churchill.

MacDermot, V. (1960). *Brain*, **83**, 24.

McEntee, W. J., and Mancall, E. L. (1965). *Neurology (Minneapolis)*, **15**, 69.

McPherson, A. (1967). *J. Physiol. (Lond.)*, **188**, 121.

McQuillen, M. P., and Johns, R. J. (1967). *Neurology (Minneapolis)*, **17**, 527.

Mellick, R. S., Mahler, R. F., and Hughes, B. P. (1962). *Lancet*, **1**, 1045.

Milhorat, A. T., Shafiq, S. A., and Goldstone, L. (1966). *Ann. N.Y. Acad. Sci.*, **138**, 246.

Milhorat, A. T., and Wolff, H. G. (1943). *Acta Neurol. Psychiat. (Chic.)*, **49**, 641.

Mommaerts, W. F. H. M., Illingworth, B., Pearson, C. M., Guillory, R. J., and Seraydarian, K. (1959). *Proc. nat. Acad. Sci. (Wash.)*, **45**, 791.

Morton, N. E., and Chung, C. S. (1959). *Amer. J. hum. Genet.*, **11**, 360.

Mulder, D. W., Bastron, J. A., and Lambert, E. H. (1956). *Neurology (Minneapolis)*, **6**, 627.

Müller, R., and Kugelberg, E. (1959). *J. Neurol. Neurosurg. Psychiat.*, **22**, 314.

Munsat, T. L. (1967). *Neurology (Minneapolis)*, **17**, 359

Murphy, E. G., Thompson, M. W., Corey, P. N. J., and Conen, P. E. (1965). In *Muscle*, ed. W. M. Paul, E. E. Daniel, C. M. Kay, and G. Monckton. Oxford, Pergamon Press.

Nattrass, F. J. (1954). *Brain*, **77**, 549.

Nissen, K. (1923). *Z. klin. Med.*, **97**, 58.

Okinaka, S., Shizume, K., Iino, S., Watanabe, A., Irie, M., Noguchi, A., Kuma, S., Kuma, K., and Ito, T. (1957). *J. clin. Endocr.*, **17**, 1454.

Oosterhuis, H. J. G. H., Van der Geld, H., Feltkamp, T. E. W., and Peetoom, F. (1964). *J. Neurol. Neurosurg. Psychiat.*, **27**, 345.

Oppenheim, H. (1900). *Mschr. Psychiat. Neurol.*, **8**, 233.

Osserman, K. E. (1958). *Myasthenia Gravis.* New York, Grune & Stratton.

Osserman, K. E., and Kaplan, L. I. (1953). *Arch. Neurol. Psychiat. (Chic.)*, **70**, 385.

Paine, R. S. (1963). *Develop. Med. Child Neurol.*, **5**, 115.

Paulley, J. W., and Hughes, J. P. (1960). *Brit. med. J.*, **2**, 1562.

Pearce, G. W. (1964). Chapter 9, *Disorders of Voluntary Muscle*, ed. J. N. Walton. London, Churchill.

Pearce, J. M. S., Pennington, R. J. T., and Walton, J. N. (1964). *J. Neurol. Neurosurg. Psychiat.*, **27**, 96.

Pearson, C. M. (1957). *New Engl. J. Med.*, **256**, 1069.

Pearson, C. M. (1962). *Brain*, **85**, 109.

Pearson, C. M. (1964). Chapter 12, *Disorders of Voluntary Muscle*, ed. J. N. Walton. London, Churchill.

Pearson, C. M. (1966). *Ann. N.Y. Acad. Sci.*, **138**, 293.

Pearson, C. M., and Rose, A. S. (1960). *Res. Publ. Ass. nerv. ment. Dis.*, **38**, 422.

Pennington, R. J. T. (1965). Chapter 2, *Biochemical Aspects of Neurological Disorders*, ed. J. N. Cumings and M. Kremer. Oxford, Blackwell.

Perkoff, G. T., Silber, R., Tyler, F. H., Cartwright, G. E., and Wintrobe, M. M. (1959). *Amer. J. Med.*, **26**, 891.

Philip, U., Walton, J. N., and Smith, C. A. B. (1956). *Ann. hum. Genet.*, **21**, 155.

Poskanzer, D. C., and Kerr, D. N. S. (1961a). *Lancet*, **2**, 511.

Poskanzer, D. C., and Kerr, D. N. S. (1961b). *Amer. J. Med.*, **31**, 328.

Price, H. M., Gordon, G. B., Pearson, C. M., Munsat, T. L., and Blumberg, J. M. (1965). *Proc. nat. Acad. Sci. (Wash.)*, **54**, 1398.

PRINEAS, J. W., HALL, R., and BARWICK, D. D. (1968). *Quart. J. Med.*, in the press.

PRINEAS, J. W., MASON, A. S., and HENSON, R. A. (1965). *Brit. med. J.*, **1**, 1034.

PRUZANSKI, W. (1966). *Brain*, **89**, 563.

REFSUM, S., LOUNUM, A., SJAASTAD, O., and ENGESET, A. (1967). *Neurology (Minneapolis)*, **17**, 345.

RICHTERICH, R., ROSIN, S., AEBI, U., and ROSSI, E. (1963). *Amer. J. hum. Genet.*, **15**, 133.

ROMANUL, F. C. A. (1966). *Nature (Lond.)*, **212**, 1369.

ROSE, A. L., and WALTON, J. N. (1966). *Brain*, **89**, 747.

ROSMAN, N. P., and KAKULAS, B. A. (1966). *Brain*, **89**, 769.

ROWLAND, L. P. (1955). *Neurology (Minneapolis)*, **5**, 612.

ROWLAND, L. P., and ESKENAZI, A. N. (1956). *Neurology (Minneapolis)*, **6**, 667.

SCHAPIRA, F., DREYFUS, J. C., SCHAPIRA, G., and DEMOS, J. (1960). *Rev. franc. Etud. clin. biol.*, **5**, 990.

SCHMID, R., and HAMMAKER, L. (1961). *New Engl. J. Med.*, **264**, 223.

SCHMID, R., and MAHLER, R. (1959). *J. clin. Invest.*, **38**, 2044.

SCHWAB, R. S. and LELAND, C. C. (1953). *J. Amer. med. Ass.*, **153**, 1270.

SHORT, J. K. (1963). *Neurology (Minneapolis)*, **13**, 526.

SHY, G. M. (1960). *Res. Publ. Ass. nerv. ment. Dis.*, **38**, 274.

SHY, G. M. (1962). *Wld. Neurol.*, **3**, 149.

SHY, G. M., (1966). In *Symposium über progressive Muskeldystrophie*, ed. E. Kuhn. Berlin, Heidelberg, New York, Springer-Verlag.

SHY, G. M., ENGEL, W. K., SOMERS, J. E., and WANKO, T. (1963). *Brain*, **86**, 793.

SHY, G. M., and GONATAS, N. K. (1964). *Science*, **145**, 493.

SHY, G. M., GONATAS, N. K., and PEREZ, M. C. (1966). *Brain*, **89**, 133.

SHY, G. M., and MAGEE, K. R. (1956). *Brain*, **79**, 610.

SHY, G. M., WANKO, T., ROWLEY, P. T., and ENGEL, A. G. (1961). *Exp. Neurol.*, **3**, 53.

SIBLEY, J. A., and LEHNINGER, A. L. (1949). *J. biol. Chem.*, **177**, 859.

SILVESTRI, T. (1909). *Gazz. Osp. Clin.*, **30**, 577.

SIMPSON, J. A. (1958). *Brain*, **81**, 112.

SIMPSON, J. A. (1960). *Scot. med. J.*, **5**, 419.

SIMPSON, J. A. (1964). Chapter 13, *Disorders of Voluntary Muscle*, ed. J. N. Walton. London, Churchill.

SIMPSON, J. A. (1965). Chapter 3, *Biochemical Aspects of Neurological Disorders*, ed. J. N. Cumings and M. Kremer. Oxford, Blackwell.

SIMPSON J. A. (1966). *Ann. N.Y. Acad. Sci.*, **135**, 506.

SKYRING, A. P., and MCKUSICK, V. A. (1961). *Amer. J. med. Sci.*, **242**, 534.

SMITH, J. B., and PATEL, A. (1965). *Neurology (Minneapolis)*, **15**, 469.

SPILLER, W. G. (1913). *Brain*, **36**, 75.

SPIRO, A. J., SHY, G. M., and GONATAS, N. K. (1966). *Arch. Neurol. (Chic.)*, **14**, 1.

STEINERT, H. (1909). *Dtsch. Z. Nervenheilk.*, **37**, 58.

STEPHENS, J., and LEWIN, E. (1965). *J. Neurol. Neurosurg. Psychiat.*, **28**, 104.

STERN, G., ROSE, A. L., and JACOBS, K. (1967). *J. Neurol. Sci.*, in the press.

STEVENSON, A. C. (1953). *Ann. Eugen. (Lond.)*, **18**, 50.

STRAUSS, A. J. L., SEEGAL, B. C., HSU, K. C., BURKHOLDER, P. M., NASTUK, W. L., and OSSERMAN, K. E. (1960). *Proc. Soc. exp. Biol. (N.Y.)*, **105**, 184.

STRAUSS, A. J. L., SMITH, C. W., CAGE, G. W., VAN DER GELD, H. W. R., MCFARLIN, D. E., and BARLOW, M. (1966). *Ann. N.Y. Acad. Sci.*, **135**, 557.

TARUI, S., OKUNO, G., IKURA, Y., TANAKA, T., SUDA, M., and NISHIKAWA, M. (1965). *Biochem. Biophys. Res. Comm.*, **19**, 517.

THOMASEN, E. (1948). *Myotonia—Thomsen's Disease (Myotonia Congenita), Paramyotonia, Dystrophia Myotonica.* Aarhus, Universitetsforlaget.

THOMSEN, J. (1876). *Arch. Psychiat. Nervenkr.*, **6**, 706.

THOMAS, W. H. S., LEYBURN, P., and WALTON, J. N. (1960). *Brit. med. J.*, **2**, 1276.

THOMSON, W. H. S., MACLAURIN, J. C., and PRINEAS, J. W. (1963). *J. Neurol. Neurosurg. Psychiat.*, **26**, 60.

TODD, J. W. (1961). *Lancet*, **2**, 1111.

TYLER, F. H., STEPHENS, F. E., GUNN, F. D., and PERKOFF, G. T. (1951). *J. clin. Invest.*, **30**, 492.

TYLER, F. H., and WINTROBE, M. M. (1950). *Ann. intern. Med.*, **32**, 72.

VAN DEN BOSCH, J. (1963). In *Research in Muscular Dystrophy*, p. 23. London, Pitman.

VAN DER GELD, H. W. R., and STRAUSS, A. J. L. (1966). *Lancet*, **1**, 57.

VAN DER MEULEN, J. P., GILBERT, G. J., and KANE, C. A. (1961). *New Engl. J. Med.*, **264**, 1.

VANIER, T. M. (1960). *Brit. med. J.*, **2**, 1284.

VAN'T HOFF, W. (1962). *Quart. J. Med.*, **31**, 385.

VICTOR, M., HAYES, R., and ADAMS, R. D. (1962). *New Engl. J. Med.*, **267**, 1267.

WALSH, F. B. (1957). *Clinical Neuro-ophthalmology*, 2nd edition. London, Bailliere, Tindall & Cox.

WALTON, J. N. (1952). *J. Neurol. Neurosurg. Psychiat.*, **15**, 219.

WALTON, J. N. (1955). *Ann. hum. Genet.*, **20**, 1.

WALTON, J. N. (1956a). *Ann. hum. Genet.*, **21**, 40.

WALTON, J. N. (1956b). *Lancet*, **1**, 1023.

WALTON, J. N. (1957). *J. Neurol. Neurosurg. Psychiat.*, **20**, 144.

WALTON, J. N. (1960). *Res. Publ. Ass. nerv. ment. Dis.*, **38**, 378.

WALTON, J. N. (1963). Chapter 7, *Muscular Dystrophy in Man and Animals*, ed. G. H. Bourne and M. N. Golarz. Basel, Karger.

WALTON, J. N. (1964a). *Brit. med. J.*, **1**, 1271, 1344.

WALTON, J. N. (1964b). Chapter 11, *Disorders of Voluntary Muscle*, ed. J. N. Walton. London, Churchill.

WALTON, J. N. (1965a). Chapter 1, *Biochemical Aspects of Neurological Disorders*, ed. J. N. Cumings and M. Kremer. Oxford, Blackwell.

WALTON, J. N. (1965b). In *Muscle*, ed. W. M. Paul, E. E. Daniel, C. M. Kay, and G. Monckton. Oxford, Pergamon Press.

WALTON, J. N. (1966). *Abstracts of World Medicine*, **40**, 1, 81.

WALTON, J. N., and ADAMS, R. D. (1958). *Polymyositis.* Edinburgh, Livingstone.

WALTON, J. N., GESCHWIND, N., and SIMPSON, J. A. (1956). *J. Neurol. Neurosurg. Psychiat.*, **19**, 224.

WALTON, J. N., and NATTRASS, F. J. (1954). *Brain*, **77**, 169.

WALTON, J. N., and WARRICK, C. K. (1954). *Brit. J. Radiol.*, **27**, 1.

WELANDER, L. (1951). *Acta med. Scand.*, Suppl. 265, 1.

WELANDER, L. (1957). *Acta genet. (Basel)*, **7**, 321.

WELANDER, L. (1966). In *Symposium über progressive Muskeldystrophie*, ed. E. Kuhn. Berlin, Heidelberg, New York, Springer-Verlag.

WHITE, R. G., and MARSHALL, A. H. E. (1962). *Lancet*, **2**, 120.

WIEME, R. J., and HERPOL, J. E. (1962). *Nature (Lond.)*, **194**, 287.

WILLISON, R. G. (1965). *Proc. 6th int. Congr. EEG clin. Neurophysiol.*, p. 711.

WILSON, J., and WALTON, J. N. (1959). *J. Neurol. Neurosurg. Psychiat.*, **22**, 320.

WOCHNER, R. D., DREWS, G., STROBER, W., and WALDMANN, T. A. (1966). *J. clin. Invest.*, **45**, 321.

ZELLWEGER, H., BROWN, B. I., McCORMICK, W. F., and TU, J. B. (1965). *Ann. pædiat.*, **205**, 413.

ZIERLER, K. L., and ANDRES, R. (1957). *J. clin. Invest.*, **36**, 730.

CHAPTER 5

DISORDERS OF CEREBRAL CIRCULATION

The late LORD BRAIN

CEREBRAL ISCHÆMIA DUE TO ATHEROMA

DURING recent years, a large amount of work has been done on the effects of atheroma on the cerebral circulation. This growing interest may be due partly to the fact that the incidence of cerebral ischæmia has been rising in Great Britain while that of cerebral hæmorrhage has been falling. Yates (1964) has analyzed the Registrar General's figures and reviewed the necropsy reports in the case of 3,397 fatal "strokes" occurring in the three largest Manchester hospitals. He found that in the 1930's cerebral hæmorrhage was nearly three times as common a cause of death as cerebral infarction but during the last five years cerebral infarction has become the commoner. This change of pattern is partly due to the gradual fall in the number of deaths from cerebral hæmorrhage and partly to an abrupt rise in the cases of cerebral infarction which started about 1947 and ceased about 1955. In the thirty year period under review, death from cerebral hæmorrhage has been equally common in men and women at almost all ages, but in people of equivalent age, cerebral infarction has always been more common in men. Analysis of the figures by age and by cohorts shows a relative reduction of deaths from cerebral infarction during the war period (1940–45) and this reduction was proportionately similar in all age groups prone to the disease. Yates suggests that this fact is most easily explained if cerebral infarction is the result of two conditions—an underlying narrowing of the arteries by atherosclerosis, which steadily progresses with increasing age, and added complications, such as thrombosis. The complications, which are often the immediate cause of death, appear to have been reduced by some factor which existed during the war period, possibly dietetic restriction.

The Site of the Atheroma Reponsible for Cerebral Infarction

Until comparatively recently, the attention of pathologists in cases of cerebral infarction was directed to the state of the intracranial arteries. Hutchinson and Yates (1956) in a classical paper studied the effects of atheroma of the vertebral artery in its cervical portion. They found that this was frequently associated with atheroma of the carotid artery at the sinus and suggested that since the carotid and vertebral arteries were collateral channels, each capable up to a point of supplying the deficiencies of the other through the circle of Willis, stenosis of the vertebral arteries might play an important part in the development of certain symptoms associated with occlusion of the internal carotid arteries. They drew attention to distortion of the vertebral arteries caused by osteophytes in the spine in cervical spondylosis and they reported 4 cases of cerebellar infarction, in all of which both the vertebral and the carotid arteries were stenosed by atheroma and in each of which an infarct of one or other cerebrellar hemisphere was present.

More recently, Yates and Hutchinson (1961) have published a study of the role of stenosis of the extracranial cerebral arteries in cerebral infarction. They made a full post-mortem examination of 100 cases of clinically diagnosed cerebral ischæmia, including a detailed study by dissection and histological examination of the whole course of both vertebral and both carotid arteries. Cerebral infarction was found in 35 cases in which there were in all 74 separate infarcts. Only 22 of the infarcts in 19 of the cases were associated with significant stenosis or occlusion of intracranial arteries, but in all except 3 of the 35 cases there was significant stenosis or occlusion of extracranial cerebral arteries. The lesions in the abnormal vessels were due mainly to atheroma and thrombosis, and hæmorrhage was found in the atheromatous plaques in many cases.

There was serious stenosis or occlusion of both internal carotid and vertebral arteries in 33 of the 100 cases, of the internal carotid arteries alone in 18 cases and of the vertebral arteries alone in 7. The internal carotid arteries were severely affected in 51 cases, 77 vessels being involved, in 67 of which the site of disease was at the carotid sinus. Among the 40 cases of serious vertebral stenosis or occlusion the disease was rather more widely distributed along the vessel, though in 36 of the 57 severely affected arteries, the stenosis was in the first 2 cm.

It follows from studies such as this that if a patient is suspected of cerebral ischæmia due to atheroma, the condition of the extracranial arteries, carotids and vertebrals, needs to be taken into account as well as that of their intracranial branches.

The Pathogenesis of Cerebral Ischæmia Associated with Atheroma

It is perhaps natural to suppose that narrowing of major vessels such as the internal carotid and vertebral arteries by atheroma is sufficient in itself to explain cerebral ischæmia leading to infarction. Brice, Dowsett and Lowe (1964), however, having studied the hæmodynamic effects of carotid artery stenosis, have shown that a very severe degree of narrowing is necessary in order to reduce the blood flow. For example, if the minimal area of cross-section of a vessel is more than 5 square mm. the blood flow will not be reduced even by long stenosis or by several stenoses in series. If the minimal area is between 2 and 5 square mm. the blood flow may be reduced, depending on the shape, on the number of stenoses in series, and to a less extent, on the length of the stenoses. Cerebral infarction, however, certainly occurs in the absence of the critical degree of narrowing necessary to reduce the blood flow according to Brice and his colleagues.

The blood flow through a vessel depends not only upon the calibre of the vessel but also upon the blood pressure available to drive the blood through it. Hutchinson and Yates (1956) stressed the importance of systemic circulatory factors in the production of cerebral ischæmia. Cerebral atheroma and coronary atheroma are often associated and the hypotension resulting from an attack of coronary thrombosis may in turn precipitate an episode of cerebral ischæmia. Hutchinson and Yates found 22 cases of severe coronary atherosclerosis, including 7 with myocardial infarction, and among the 22 were 13 cases of cerebral infarction. Shock from any cause may have the same effect in the elderly—for example a surgical operation, especially one conducted under induced hypotension. In their series, Hutchinson and Yates had 11 patients who died after surgical operation (3 with cerebral infarction) and 6 following traumatic shock (2 with cerebral infarction). Anæmia may also be a potent factor in impairing cerebral metabolism, especially when associated with vascular stenosis and hypotension. Moreover, as Hutchinson and Yates point out, intermittent hypotension may itself be the result of arterial disease, for example, through interference with the carotid sinus reflex or other baroreceptor mechanism. Whether vasospasm plays any part, save in exceptional circumstances, is uncertain.

THE SUBCLAVIAN "STEAL" SYNDROME

The subclavian "steal" or "brachio-basilar insufficiency" syndrome, recently described, is the result of unilateral occlusion of the first part of the subclavian artery before the origin of the vertebral artery. The effect of this is that when the pulseless limb is exercised blood flows down the vertebral artery on the affected side, to supply the subclavian artery beyond the obstruction, and may thus indirectly cause symptoms of ischæmia within the vertebrobasilar distribution, such as vertigo, syncope, or transitory blindness. Cases have been described by North, Fields, DeBakey and Crawford (1962) and by Siekert, Millikan and Whisnant (1964). Cameron and Wright (1964) report an interesting single case of olfactory hallucinations as a symptom of the subclavian "steal" syndrome. The obstruction was to the left subclavian artery and the symptoms were relieved by ligature of the left vertebral artery. Presumably in this case, the ischæmia lay within the distribution of the branches of the posterior cerebral arteries going to the temporal lobes.

The Effects of Head Movement on the Cerebral Circulation

Attention was first attracted to the possible influence of cervical spondylosis on the cerebral circulation by the work of Hutchinson and Yates (1956). "We would stress", they wrote, "the intimate relationship the vertebral artery bears on its medial aspect to the neurocentral joint within the vertebral canal, and the fact that it is at this point that the artery passes immediately anterior to the emerging cervical nerve root, each root being supplied by a small arterial twig. This anatomical relationship assumes importance when the cervical vertebræ are affected by degenerative osteoarthritic change; this condition was present in several of the specimens we examined." That the neurocentral joint is frequently affected in cervical spondylosis was emphasized by Pallis, Jones and Spillane (1954). "The bony prominence which develops displaces the artery laterally and in the more severe cases in an anterior direction also. The displacement so produced varies from a gentle curve . . . to a marked distortion." It was important to establish, as the work of Hutchinson and Yates did, that even with the neck at rest in the forward facing position cervical spondylosis could substantially interfere with the circulation through the vertebral arteries. But the neck is rarely at rest for long during waking life: it is the site of frequent movements, (lateral rotation, flexion and extension) and to understand the full extent of the possible effects of cervical spondylosis upon the cerebral blood flow it is necessary to begin by reviewing what is known about the influence of neck movements upon the cerebral circulation, both in normal people and in patients suffering from cervical spondylosis.

de Kleyn (1939) in a study of positional nystagmus investigated the influence of head posture on the blood flow through the vertebral arteries. He ran fluid through the vertebral arteries of cadavers, and showed that rotation of the head to one side abolished the flow through the opposite vertebral artery. He attributed this to what he called the curious course of the vertebral artery between the atlas and the skull, the obstruction occurring at that site when the head was rotated. He added that although in man the auditory artery normally arises from the basilar artery it may arise from the vertebral. Discussing the collateral supply to the basilar artery he pointed out that obstruction of one vertebral artery would normally cause no symptoms of basilar insufficiency, but one vertebral artery may be very small, as in one case in his series, and if so, and the other is obstructed, the supply to the basilar artery from the vertebrals would be entirely cut off. He thought that, when the auditory artery comes off the vertebral, obstruction of the latter might explain positional nystagmus and vertigo. Tatlow and Bammer (1957) were led by the clinical observation that neurological symptoms could be produced by head-turning to study the effects of head rotation upon the vertebral arteries, and, like de Kleyn, they showed in the cadaver that rotation of the head to one side produced narrowing of the opposite vertebral artery at the atlanto-axial level.

Toole and Tucker (1960) have studied the influence of the position of the head upon the cerebral circulation. In 20 human cadavers they observed the flow of fluid through the two carotid and two vertebral arteries in relation to the position of the head. It is noteworthy that in three instances one vertebral artery was congenitally so small that no flow could be established in it. Their observations showed that on changing the position of the head flow stopped in one or other, or sometimes both, vertebral arteries in 90 per cent of cases and in one or other, or sometimes both internal carotids, in 85 per cent of cases. Rotation of the head was the movement by far the most likely to interrupt the flow in either vessel. Rotation to one side might interrupt the flow in the ipsilateral or contralateral vertebral artery, rather more frequently in the latter, but in the case of the carotid artery with one exception it was the ipsilateral vessel which was compressed. Toole and Tucker note that compression of the carotid artery may occur against the transverse process of the atlas, as postulated by Boldrey *et al.* (1956), and cause distortion of the vertebral artery as it lies upon the atlas. Finally, they say: "The degree of head-turning necessary to impair the vertebral flow may be small if, in addition to arterio-sclerotic plaques and loss of vascular elasticity, there is cervical osteoarthritis, the osteophytes projecting from the apophyseal and uncovertebral joints into the lumen of the transverse foramina. These protuberances produce vessel distortion and compression, which varies during movement of the cervical spine."

Maslowski (1960) using angiography to investigate the cerebral circulation in patients suspected of intracranial lesions, has confirmed that the lumen of the atlanto-axial segment of the vertebral artery may be narrowed, or temporarily occluded, in full rotation of the head to the opposite side, and his studies also suggested that the vertebral artery in its intraspinal course can be constricted by the joints of the cervical spine in middle-aged individuals when the head is rotated towards the side of the artery. Bauer, Sheehan, Wechsler and Meyer (1962) and Bauer, Wechsler and Meyer (1961), using angiography, have not only confirmed that in the presence of cervical spondylosis rotation of the head to one side may cause narrowing of the ipsilateral vertebral artery in its intraspinal course, but also have shown that the same vessel may appear normal in calibre if the angiogram is done with the head in the forward-looking position, or rotated to the contralateral side. Maslowski (1961) states that flexion of the neck may also cause impairment of filling of the lower part of the vertebral artery. These observations show that rotation of the head to one side may in normal individuals impair, or temporarily abolish, the blood flow through the atlantoaxial segment of the ipsilateral vertebral artery, while in the presence of cervical spondylosis it may have the same effect upon the intra-spinal course of the contralateral vertebral artery.

In these circumstances the cerebral circulation must depend upon the internal carotid arteries, so it is important to know what is happening to them. It has been shown by Boldrey et al. (1956), and Hardesty et al. (1960), that head rotation may lead to reduction of blood flow in the contralateral internal carotid artery by compression of this vessel against the lateral process of the atlas. Bauer, Sheehan, Wechsler and Meyer (1962) have confirmed this, showing by angiography, that rotation of the head may lead not only to compression of the contralateral internal carotid artery against the lateral process of the atlas, but also to kinking and stenosis of a tortuous internal carotid artery in its cervical portion on head rotation to either the ipsilateral or the contralateral side.

During recent years the compensatory value of the mutually collateral blood supply through carotids and vertebrals to the circle of Willis has been increasingly recognized, and it is especially well illustrated by the observations of Hutchinson and Yates that in the presence of atheroma of both carotids and vertebrals, occlusion of one carotid artery could lead to infarction of the cerebellum. The dynamic aspect of these complex interrelationships has recently been studied by Bauer, Wechsler, and Meyer (1961). These workers made electroencephalographic studies of patients during unilateral carotid compression alone, and unilateral carotid compression combined with rotation of the head to the opposite side. They studied eighteen patients, seventeen of whom had vertebro-basilar insufficiency proved by bilateral carotid and vertebral angiograms. In their series no electroencephalographic changes occurred with hyperextension of the neck, hyperextension with turning of the head to the left or right, or with head turning alone. Seven of the eighteen patients had a positive carotid compression test, consisting of induction of electroencephalographic changes, and four of these showed further electroencephalographic changes over the affected hemisphere when head rotation to one side was added to digital compression of the carotid artery. The authors concluded that the additional changes produced by head rotation must have been due to vertebral artery compression.

A further factor which needs to be considered as a possible cause of cerebral symptoms produced by rotation of the head is carotid sinus sensitivity. This question is considered by Bauer, Wechsler and Meyer, who after reviewing the literature, and themselves making observations, conclude that compression of the carotid sinus could not be responsible for the electro-encephalographic changes which occurred on head rotation.

These observations, together with other recent additions to our knowledge of the cerebral circulation as a whole, show that the blood flow through the nervous structures of the posterior fossa depends upon a number of factors.

1. The relative size of the vertebral arteries, since, if one is much larger than the other, obstruction of the larger one will have disproportionately severe effects. Hutchinson and Yates (1956) comment on the variation in the size of the vertebral arteries, saying: "The variations we found were of the same order as those described by Stopford (1916) who in 150 specimens found the left to be the larger in 51 per cent, the right the larger in 41 per cent and the arteries of equal size in only 8 per cent."

2. The blood flow through either or both vertebral arteries may be diminished by arterial disease, especially atheroma, at any point in their course.

3. Compression of either or both vessels from outside may reduce blood flow especially in cervical spondylosis.

4. The effects of diminution of the blood flow through one or both vertebral arteries will be influenced by the condition of the collateral circulation. This, again, may be the site of congenital abnormalities, a small posterior communicating artery on one or both sides being particularly important.

5. Atheroma of one or both internal carotid arteries, or common carotid arteries, by impeding the collateral blood supply may intensify the effects of vertebrobasilar ischæmia.

6. As already described, neck movements may in a complex fashion cause temporary diminution in the blood flow through either the vertebral or the internal carotid arteries, or both especially in the presence of cervical spondylosis.

7. The systemic blood pressure is of fundamental importance as the ultimate source of the blood flow, and the fact that it may be reflexly disturbed through the activity of the carotid sinus has already been mentioned. Other factors influencing the systemic blood pressure will have to be considered in relation to diagnosis.

8. The vertebrobasilar blood supply will also be influenced by substances which produce vasodilatation of cerebral vessels, such as CO_2 and more indirectly by factors influencing blood volume, hæmoglobin content, etc.

To sum up these observations, then, we may say that either lateral rotation or extension of the neck may, in certain circumstances, cause temporary impairment, or even complete abolition of the blood flow through one or both vertebral arteries, and may even also impair the circulation through one internal carotid artery. Pathologically we are dealing with two variables, cervical spondylosis causing compression by osteophytes in the neighbourhood of one or both vertebral arteries, and atheroma of the vertebrobasilar system and internal carotid arteries which naturally renders them more vulnerable to the effects of pressure. At one extreme it is certainly possible for severe cervical spondylosis to lead to vascular symptoms in the absence of atheroma, though for various reasons this is uncommon. At the other extreme some at least of the symptoms of intermittent vertebrobasilar ischæmia may be due to atheroma in the absence of cervical spondylosis, but in many cases both factors are present.

The Transient Ischæmic Attack

There is an episodic form of cerebral ischæmia the cause of which has given rise to much discussion. This is the transient ischæmic attack, an episode of transient but recurrent ischæmia repeatedly producing exactly the same symptoms, and therefore, presumably, located in the same and often small area of the brain. Denny-Brown (1951) suggested that transient ischæmic attacks might be due to the general fall in cerebral blood flow to which the narrowing of a particular vessel renders it more vulnerable than the rest. However, Marshall and Kendall (1963) studied the effect of lowering the blood pressure in patients who were subject to transient ischæmic attacks and found they could not, in such patients, produce focal symptoms before those of general cerebral ischæmia. It seems to follow that a fall in cerebral blood flow is not in general the cause of general ischæmic attacks. Fisher (1958) and Russell (1961, 1963) have observed patients during transient attacks of monocular blindness associated with atheroma and seen small white or yellow bodies passing along the retinal arteries, and it has been established by autopsy examination that these bodies may consist either of platelets (MacBryan, Bradley and Ashton, 1963) or cholesterolesters (David, Klintworth, Friedberg and Dillon, 1963). Gunning, Pickering, Robb-Smith and Russell (1964) have observed six patients who had attacks of monocular blindness with or without contralateral hemiplegia. In some cases they observed white or yellow bodies in the retinal arteries during the attacks of blindness and all patients had stenosis of the internal carotid artery with thrombi composed of fibrin, platelets and leucocytes at the site of the stenosis. All these observations suggest that transient ischæmic attacks may be due to emboli of this kind lodging at a point in a cerebral artery already narrowed by atheroma, and producing transient ischæmic symptoms before breaking up and passing on. It is doubtful, however, whether every case of transient ischæmic attack is to be explained in this way. If such small emboli are being discharged into the internal carotid artery on one side why should they repeatedly lodge at the same site, unless perhaps because there is atheromatous narrowing there. It may well be that not all transient ischæmic attacks are due to the same cause and possibly in some cases, at least, when there is already atheromatous narrowing of a cerebral artery, vasodilatation in surrounding areas may temporarily compete for blood with the affected vessel, as a result of which the circulation to it may diminish because, owing to its atheromatous narrowing, it is unable to dilate normally.

PROGNOSIS AND SURVIVAL IN HEMIPLEGIA

Adams and Merrett (1961) have studied the factors influencing the prognosis and survival in a group of 736 hemiplegics, admitted to the geriatric wards of the Belfast City Hospital between 1948 and 1956. 26 patients were untraced, leaving 710 for study.

They classified their patients in three groups:

1. Recovered, further divided into two grades, grade I, those who became fully independent with normal intellect and some use of the affected hand and ability to walk with confidence, grade II, patients who became able to walk but were handicapped by a useless arm and needed help with dressing and toilet. Some had impaired intellect but none were incontinent.

2. Long-stay, those who failed to improve appreciably after at least three months of intensive treatment, becoming chair-fast or bed-fast, and incapable of walking alone. They were usually confused and incontinent.

3. Died, those who died within two months of onset before the likely response to treatment could be assessed.

81 per cent of these 710 patients survived two months but among those who survived the chance of being able to move about and look after themselves was only slightly better than that of being permanently incapacitated (42·3 per cent compared with 38·5 per cent). There was no difference between men and women. Older patients were found to be more likely to be permanently incapacitated, but age in itself did not preclude a good recovery, nor did a lesion of the dominant hemisphere.

Men and women who recovered lived longer than those who became long-stay patients. For technical reasons, average survival for the whole series could not be estimated. However, it was possible to assess the half-way mark with reasonable accuracy—that is, the number of years after a stroke which half of a given group might expect to live (or, conversely, the number of years which would be exceeded by less than half of a group). Comparing these figures with the normal life expectation of persons of the same age, the group half-survivals were much less than the normal expectation but showed that 50 per cent of the patients of either sex who recovered from their strokes survived at least six years if aged less than 65 at the onset, or about $3\frac{1}{2}$ years if men or 4 years if women, over that age. This was considerably better than the survival in the long-stay patients who had not recovered.

Adams and Hurwitz (1963) investigated the mental factors which impede recovery from strokes, in 45 long-stay hemiplegic invalids. 18 patients, (40 per cent) had severe residual paralysis and sensory deficit with varying degrees of intellectual impairment. They appeared to have had extensive infarction in the distribution of the middle cerebral artery. 6 of these showed evidence of neglect of the affected limbs and some denied that they were in any way abnormal. Two men had severe motor apraxia and 7 patients had postural imbalance attributed to vertebrobasilar insufficiency. Three patients simply refused to try. The authors conclude that half of these chronic invalids had mental barriers—defects of cerebral function other than paralysis or a florid psychosis—to account for their lack of response to long-continued efforts to restore activity. Other such factors mentioned in the discussion include loss of recent memory and true depression.

References

ADAMS, G. F., and HURWITZ, L. J. (1963). *Lancet*, **2**, 533.

ADAMS, G. F., and MERRETT, J. D. (1961). *Brit. med. J.*, **1**, 309.

BAUER, R. B., SHEEHAN, S., WECHSLER, N., and MEYER, J. S. (1962). *Neuorology (Minneap.)*, **12**, 698.

BAUER, R. B., WECHSLER, N., and MEYER, J. S. (1961). *Ann. intern. Med.*, **55**, 283.

BOLDREY, E., MAASS, L., and MILLER, E. R. (1956). *J. Neurosurg.*, **13**, 127.

BRICE, J. G., DOWSETT, D. J., and LOWE, R. D. (1964). *Brit. med. J.*, **2**, 1363.

CAMERON, D. J., and WRIGHT, I. S. (1964). *Ann. intern. Med.*, **61**, 128.

DAVID, N. J., KLINTWORTH, G. K., FRIEDBERG, S. J., and DILLON, M. (1963). *Neurology (Minneap.)*, **13**, 708.

DENNY-BROWN, D. (1951). *Med. Clin. N. Amer.*, **35**, 1457.

DIMANT, S. (1959). *Brit. J. Surg.*, **46**, 333.

FISHER, C. M. (1958). *Neurology* **9**, 333.

GUNNING, A. J., PICKERING, G. W., ROBB SMITH, A. H. T., and RUSSELL, R. W. (1964). *Quart. J. Med.*, **33**, 158.

HARDESTY, W. H., ROBERTS, B., TOOLE, J. F., and ROYSTER, H. P. (1960). *New. Engl. J. Med.*, **263**, 744.

HUTCHINSON, E. C., and YATES, P. O. (1956). *Brain*, **79**, 319.

DE KLEYN, A. (1939). *Confin. neurol.*, **2**, 257.

MACBRYAN, D. J., BRADLEY, R. D., and ASHTON, N. (1963). *Lancet*, **1**, 697.

MARSHALL, J., and KENDELL, R. E. (1963). *Brit. med. J.*, **2**, 1131.

MASLOWSKI, H. A. (1960). *J. Neurol. Neurosurg. Psychiat.*, **23**, 355.

MASLOWSKI, H. A. (1961). *J. Neurol. Neurosurg. Psychiat.*, **24**, 95.

NORTH, R. R., FIELDS, W. S., DEBAKEY, M. E., and CRAWFORD, E. S. (1962). *Neurology (Minneap.)*, **12**, 810.

PALLIS, C., JONES, A. M., and SPILLANE, J. D. (1954). *Brain*, **77**, 274.

RUSSELL, R. W. (1961). *Lancet*, **2**, 1422.

RUSSELL, R. W. (1963). *Lancet*, **2**, 1354.

SIEKERT, R. G., MILLIKAN, C. H., and WHISNANT, J. P. (1964). *J. Amer. med. Ass.*, **176**, 19.

STOPFORD, J. S. B. (1916). *J. Anat. Physiol.*, **51**, 250.

TATLOW, W. F. T., and BAMMER, H. G. (1957). *Neurology (Minneap.)*, **7**, 331.

TOOLE, J. F., and TUCKER, S. H. (1960). *Arch. Neurol.*, **2**, 616.

YATES, P. O. (1964). *Lancet*, **1**, 65.

YATES, P. O., and HUTCHINSON, E. C. (1961). *Spec. Rep. Ser. med. Res. Coun. (Lond.)*, No. 300, H.M. Stationery Office.

CHAPTER 6

SURGERY OF CEREBRAL HÆMORRHAGE

R. T. Johnson

SUDDEN leakage of blood into the brain or over its surface induces changes of great complexity in cerebral function. Not infrequently these changes are so slight that they pass unnoticed or are mis-diagnosed as influenza, fibrositis or lumbago. Extensive changes in cerebral function are the result not only of focal damage by the hæmorrhage but of variation in blood flow due to arterial spasm or thrombosis, of secondary brain stem compression and distortion produced by raised intracranial pressure and of a little understood process whereby a chain reaction is set up—change of function in one basal area inducing progressive changes in others, without evidence of organic damage (Jefferson, 1951a).

The intensive observation of patients with post traumatic and post operative brain damage (where the injury is more accurately known) has enabled greater understanding of some of the sequels and a more logical attitude to be taken towards the treatment of patients who might otherwise have been regarded as beyond recovery. Coma on rare occasions may be the result of depressed function in a small region of the hypothalamic brain stem complex, and may prove to be just as reversible as less dramatic signs of cerebral dysfunction such as hemianopia. In fact an almost focal sign follow-ing some of the extensive operations for craniopharyngioma has been the occurrence of prolonged unconsciousness with eventual full recovery. Now that some of the major problems in the manage-ment of such patients have been overcome, it is by attention to the smallest details that one must look for further improvement. In-creasing experience leaves little doubt that if, from the earliest moment, every step is taken to prevent brain damage or dysfunction, useful recovery may occur even after periods of prolonged coma. For example, a patient recently suffered a devastating hæmorrhage (the third in 7 days) from a carotid aneurysm, and stopped breathing; fortunately the patient was in the ward and resuscitation was im-mediately effective. Within 24 hours the patient, although still tolerating an endotracheal tube, had recovered sufficiently to risk operation and the aneurysm was clipped. The patient's recovery was slow, she remained unconscious for four weeks, hemiplegic for two months, and at ten months she still had a severe memory loss and inability to use her legs efficiently, but steady improvement is being maintained. In this patient the immediate restoration of adequate respiratory function saved her life, and there is reason to feel that this life will be useful. Much future disability may be determined in the few moments of an inadequate airway.

Sound judgement as to when to perform an early tracheostomy (done carefully under local anæsthesia) may not only be life saving, but perhaps more important, will reduce morbidity. Further important factors are: the correct use of antibiotics, the correct management of metabolism, and perhaps to a lesser degree the skilled management of the blood pressure. Lumbar puncture is not without risk, for although drainage of cerebrospinal fluid containing blood may relieve headache and may be extremely beneficial in lowering intracranial tension, it may induce an increasing brain shift, with all the attendant consequences, if there is an intracerebral clot and/or extensive cerebral œdema, and there is some evidence that it may precipitate further hæmorrhage (Taylor, 1961). Lumbar puncture was immediately followed by the first hæmorrhage from a chiasmal aneurysm in one of my patients. Furthermore there would seem to be an increased risk of infection from lumbar puncture when blood is present in the cerebrospinal fluid. Two of my patients have died from uncontrollable meningitis, following careful diagnostic lumbar puncture, and when operation was carried out because of clinical deterioration, infection and not further hæmorrhage was demonstrated to be the cause of the change. It was striking that although antibiotics cleared the infection from the ventricles of the brain and cranial cavity, it remained active in the spinal subarachnoid space, where resolving blood clots caused loculation of cerebro-spinal fluid. In both instances diagnostic lumbar puncture had been carried out by the same referring unit, and these were the only cases of infection in a series of many hundred lumbar punctures. If a lumbar puncture has to be done, and sometimes this is essential, it seems wise to sterilize the skin with the old fashioned yet well tried tincture of iodine (which rarely causes anything but the mildest skin reaction if immediately washed off with spirit). The majority of patients admitted to my unit are not lumbar punctured, a departure from traditional routine—I would rather proceed to immediate angiography.

Some patients with intracranial hæmorrhage are not seriously ill and the treatment is uncontroversial and easy, but others involve most difficult decisions at all stages unless the surgeon is relieved of anxiety by adhering to certain set rules for the selection and management of patients. The management of such patients is clearly a personal matter and will vary from centre to centre; for this reason statistics are not easy to compare. My own patients are a mixed group, some are referred directly from their homes within a few hours of the hæmorrhage, some are referred when fully recovered for definitive treatment, and some because of recurrent hæmorrhage or deterioration due to other causes. Nearly all the patients have careful cerebral angiography under local anæsthesia on admission; sometimes, of course, the angiograms are incomplete (vertebral artery angiograms are usually done later under general anæsthesia), or are not diagnostic. This investigation provides the first basic information on which management of the case is planned, for it selects cases which can and should be treated immediately by the evacuation of blood clot and/or by the definitive treatment of a dangerous lesion, usually peripheral, and which is judged to be attainable without undue risk. Furthermore the difficult patients can be watched and treated by every available means until such time as they are fit for further angiographic studies or surgery, with the knowledge that a readily treatable lesion which could kill at any minute is not being neglected.

So far no differentiation has been made between the many causes of intracranial hæmorrhage, in fact they present similar problems, and not only may an early categorization result in the withholding of treatment, but may be misleading in that the various causes may mimic each other. However, certain clinical features which are of value in planning the care of such patients, and selecting treatment, have become apparent following the study of a large number of patients.

CEREBRAL HÆMORRHAGE

Hypertensive Cerebral Hæmorrhage typically occurs in a large overweight red faced individual who has had arterial hypertension for years. There are, perhaps, short lived prodromal symptoms, then the patient presents in deep coma, stertorous respirations and dense hemiplegia. The hæmatomas are believed to arise from diseased blood vessels and microaneurysms (Charcot and Bouchard, 1868; Green, 1930), and although this theory was questioned for many years (Ellis, 1909; Russell, 1954), it is again supported by recent work (Ross Russell, 1963; Cole and Yates, 1967). The bleeding usually, but by no means invariably, occurs in the internal capsule, producing hæmorrhages, thromboses, and softenings which extend to the vital mid-line areas bordering the 3rd ventricle. When hæmorrhages occur at this site little can be done therapeutically, but in patients with less severe hæmorrhages recovery can occasionally occur, and sometimes the patient may improve to a certain level when the condition becomes static. Aspiration of some of the blood clot through a burr hole may hasten or achieve recovery. Careful angiography under local anæsthesia may reveal the exact situation, and demonstrate the degree of cerebral shift. The position of mid-line structures may be monitored at frequent intervals by the use of ultra-sound. Many intracerebral hæmatomas of considerable size produce no mid-line shift and their presence can only be detected by the displacement of the smaller blood vessels (Fig. 5). The futility of dramatic surgery in the early stages is determined not only by the site of the damage but by the secondary changes, especially those resulting from downward displacement and distortion of the mid-brain (Johnson and Yates, 1956), and yet it would be wrong to dismiss the possible role of surgery in such patients on an initial diagnosis of intracerebral hæmorrhage. Absence of total hemiplegia in the first few hours may mean that the hæmorrhage is present in the temporal or frontal lobes, neglect of one side of the body or hemianopia that it is parieto-occipital. Such signs, and especially intervals of lightening coma, indicate a non-fatal hæmorrhage which may be successfully removed by aspiration or open operation. Intracerebral clots may be associated with periods of varying consciousness; a clinical picture well recognized as resulting from a subdural hæmatoma. A deterioration in the patient's condition does not necessarily indicate that a further hæmorrhage has occurred; it probably represents the result of a functional change in the brain stem produced by variations in blood flow. The classical changes of varying consciousness associated with a subdural effusion have been observed to occur in patients following the drainage of a subdural hæmatoma when the drainage holes have been left open; it is clear that the osmotic effect of the membrane in regulating the flow fluid in and out of the cavity can play no part at this stage, nor was it observed that the conscious level could be correlated with the distance of the cortical surfaces from the dura. Just as the compressed and distorted brain stem at a distance from the subdural hæmatoma responds critically to slight changes in blood flow, so do the areas of the brain forming the wall of the clot and which subserve vital functions. Severely compressed but just functioning areas of brain may cease to function if rapid decompression is brought about.

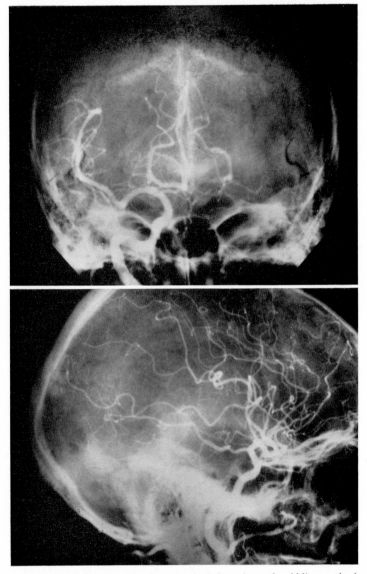

Figure 5. Angiograms showing terminal branches of middle cerebral artery displaced by occipito parietal haematoma; there is no mid line shift.

For this reason my practice has been to remove only a small amount of clot initially, and to repeat this daily or more frequently as the patient's condition indicates. Hypertensive hæmorrhages rarely occur on the brain surface, but long standing hypertension should not debar a patient from treatment if the hæmorrhage is from a treatable aneurysm, angioma, subdural hæmatoma, all of which may present with stroke-like suddenness, or is from a cerebral tumour.

Cerebral Hæmorrhage in Association with Tumours may occur into a tumour cavity or over its surface. Initially cerebral hæmorrhage with a tumour is indistinguishable from that due to other causes, although failure to improve following aspiration of blood clot or the re-collection of blood may suggest the presence of an underlying tumour. The occurrence of rapidly progressive hemiplegia over hours or days unaccompanied by headache, although in retrospect a preceeding history of fits or headache may be elicited, is character- istic of cerebral hæmorrhage with a tumour. Radioactive isotopes can be valuable in the diagnosis, perhaps, by delineating a tumour alongside an area of the hæmorrhage. The tumour is usually an astrocytoma of from Grade I to Grade III activity but one of my patients had a small left frontal meningioma some 2 cm in diameter which produced coma of stroke-like onset, with stertorous respira- tion. The coma lightened for a few days during which it was observed that, although all four limbs moved, the right side moved less well than the left. Deterioration with deepening coma produced an emergency, and an exploratory burr hole at the most likely site revealed a large hæmatoma. Partial aspiration produced improvement, and two days later a craniotomy revealed that the cause of the hæmorrhage was a torn vein on the surface of a meningioma. In retrospect the hæmorrhage was probably caused by a minor head injury.

In Summary the careful management of strokes due to hæmor- rhage may result in more complete recovery. The management entails locating the hæmorrhage and slowly draining it, eliciting the symptoms and signs that suggest pathology other than arterial disease, and taking special care of patients with strokes that present without hemiplegia.

HÆMORRHAGE DUE TO ANEURYSMS

Surgically this is by far the most important group of patients with cerebral hæmorrhage and according to Zimmerman (1963) constitutes 5 per cent of all cerebral vacular disturbance. Few problems have presented such difficulty, and such difference of opinion, so many conflicting statistics and such a wealth of literature during the past twenty years. This is perhaps understandable when one considers the complexity of the problem; the rapid developments in the surgical techniques, the deeper understanding of the pathology of aneurysm formation and life history, and the pathological effect of leakage. The challenge to surgeons was clearly indicated by Sir Charles Symonds (1924) who described a boy of 24 who died because a small aneurysm of the anterior cerebral bifurcation had ruptured, and in whom all the other arteries were healthy and no other lesion was present. He could not have chosen a better example to illustrate the problems posed by intracranial aneurysm in the ensuing years; its site, deep within the brain meant that access would have to be achieved without producing damage, and that if cure were to be attained before fatal hæmorrhage it might be necessary to operate in the presence of a brain swollen as a result of recent hæmorrhage.

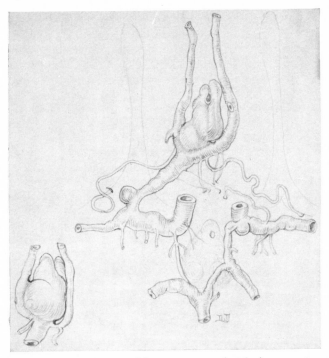

Figure 6. Multiple intracranial aneurysms; patient had no symptoms until the first and fatal subarachnoid haemorrhage from the anterior communicating aneurysmal complex.

Much of the extensive work on this type of problem has been coloured by the training, experience, and personality of the surgeon, not forgetting the skills of his associated anæsthetists, neurologists, and those from many other disciplines, that it might be helpful in the first instance to attempt to clarify the problem. Not a little of what has been devised and written about surgery of intracranial aneurysms is a solution to a particular problem of the surgeon, and this does not necessarily correspond to what might be termed the patient's problem. In the first place the leaking aneurysm may be merely an incident in extensive arterial disease or it may be part of such a comprehensive problem that surgical cure is not possible (Fig. 6). In cases of multiple aneurysm it may be difficult to know which one has bled, in spite of the indications of angiographic studies, and although as many as three and rarely four may be surgically cured, treatment is essentially a compromise. Basically, however, the problem is that a patient of virtually any age group may develop an aneurysm (incidence: 1 per cent of a population, Hanby (1952), 2 per cent, Housepian and Pool (1958). This at its simplest may be a small sac 1 cm or so in diameter arising at a vessel bifurcation, the wall containing little or no muscle and little or no elastic tissue. Such berry aneurysms are believed to arise where there are defects in the media (Eppinger, 1887; Forbus, 1930); these defects are common (80 per cent of all arteries, Carmichael, 1945), and yet aneurysms are relatively rare. The size of the defect in the media may well be a factor, for at operation such defects may be readily seen as transparent areas, perhaps 2 or 3 mm in diameter. At operation such areas are now patched with fascia, but in some of the earlier cases when their importance was not fully appreciated this was not done. Carmichael (1945) assumed that in the larger defects the internal elastic lamina was adequate, for Forbus (1930) had demonstrated the mechanical strength of the internal elastic lamina by dissection. Hackel (1927) demonstrated the progressive disruption and fragmentation of the internal elastic lamina with age, and although this is widespread and is associated with intimal hyperplasia, it might cause aneurysm formation it if occurred in relation to medial defects. There is evidence that many aneurysms, even those called vestigial (Bremer, 1943; Padget, 1948), i.e. those with a long neck and arising in the region of the origin of the posterior communicating artery, may appear in young adults with no other evidence of arteriosclerosis (Fig. 7). Walker and Allegre (1954) in a detailed study of the pathology of thirty nine aneurysms described intimal proliferation of the neck of the aneurysm, and regard this as early evidence of arteriosclerosis, if not "a disease sui generis", and noted the associated split of elastic fibres (Tuthill, 1953). Hassler (1964) found that in 17 per cent of patients presenting with an aneurysm there were associated small aneurysms, but these only occurred in patients of 30 years or over, and he suggested, therefore, that they were not congenital. He again noted intimal hypertrophy mostly on the proximal carina of arterial branches, but Pool and Potts (1965) reporting this finding state that "most aneurysms are congenital in origin, but that a few may be acquired because of arteriosclerosis." Intimal hyperplasia, however, is not arteriosclerosis

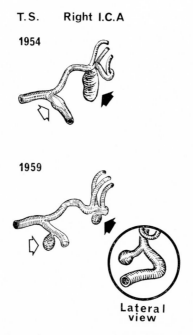

T.S.   Right I.C.A

1954

1959

Lateral
view

Figure 7. Tracings of aneurysms at intervals of 5 years. A slight fusiform swelling of the carotid has become a "vestigial" aneurysm (white arrow). An anterior communicating aneurysm which filled mainly from the left was wrapped with Terylene and the left common carotid artery was tied. When the right carotid aneurysm was clipped the anterior communicating aneurysm was observed to be firmly encased, and the angiogram showed a considerable reduction in size (black arrow.)

it occurs in areas of blood vessel walls where flow is reduced and ties in exactly with the work on fluid flow by Fox and Hugh (1966), who demonstrated that "boundary layer separation" results in areas of stasis at certain points on the vessel wall. It is interesting that these areas occur at vessel bifurcations and branches. There is such an area of stasis at the proximal carina of arterial branches which is where intimal hypertrophy is known to occur. The observations of Fox and Hugh are put forward to account for the formation of arteriosclerotic degeneration at certain points in the vessel, and there is no doubt that the areas of stasis closely correspond to reported areas of intimal hyperplasia. These hyperplastic changes which include muscle fibres and elastic fibres, as well as endothelial cells, have been observed to follow prolonged spasm, so that the "spasm" becomes permanent. Intimal hyperplasia occurs in the carotid artery following proximal ligation, and it occurs at aneurysmal necks where the boundary layer separations in a divergent stream induce stagnation at the point of divergence (Fox and Hugh, 1966). The activity of the intima may be instrumental in the safe healing of the neck of an aneurysm following the application of a clip, often inadequately placed across part of a thin walled saccule at the neck.

Virtually all large and many small aneurysms contain clot, especially after they have leaked, and this may of course be disturbed at operation producing emboli or thromboses. Clotting is not a safeguard against recurrent hæmorrhage unless an aneurysm is totally occluded, for when the neck of an aneurysm remains open the central area of clot is excavated, and, perhaps as the clot retracts, blood seeps between the clot and the wall and when it reaches a thin area further leakage will occur. Crawford (1959) deduced from an examination of pathological material that aneurysms relentlessly increase in size and rupture when they reach a diameter of about 1 cm. This finding is not supported by my clinical experience, for repeated angiograms done in many cases over a period of 20 years show that some aneurysms remain completely unchanged, while others will enlarge very considerably over a period of a few days—evidence not only of the elasticity of their walls, but suggestive that periods of activity may determine this enlargement. It is understandable that any change resulting in what might be termed trauma to part of the aneurysmal wall will provoke a cellular reaction spreading beyond the original site, resulting in progressive weakness of further areas of the wall; it is a sobering surgical experience that to dissect fully an aneurysm and then to do nothing curative is to court disaster and to risk provoking a further hæmorrhage within the next few days.

The problem posed by the aneurysm is of a ballooning area of weak vessel wall which may appear at any age; stasis at its neck will produce thickening by endothelial hyperplasia. Safe healing after the successful application of a clip is the rule, but the aneurysms must be of sufficient size to make this possible, and yet must be small enough or pliable enough (i.e. containing little or no clot) to enable dissection from the branches to be safely and adequately performed. In this, experience and surgical skill is not unimportant. In all cases the development of further aneurysms must be recognized and accepted.

The next problem is that of the subarachnoid hæmorrhage. This may not necessarily be related to the site or size of the aneurysm, and yet it is all important in the treatment of the aneurysm, for surgery carried out in the quiescent stage carries a low morbidity and mortality (5 per cent or even 1 per cent in selected series) which is quite different from that of surgery undertaken in the acute phase of the hæmorrhage especially when the patient is very ill (mortality 70 per cent for poor risk cases (Pool and Potts, 1965). Hæmorrhage is, of course, the means of diagnosing the majority of aneurysms, and its severity in an individual patient can be the compelling and cogent reason for taking risks involved in the elaborate surgery. Account must be taken also of previous slight hæmorrhages, that either did not warrant or achieve hospital admission (Symonds, 1952). Increasing awareness of the significance of slight hæmorrhages is resulting in the much earlier admission of patients to hospital and this must improve the results of both surgical and conservative treatment. But early diagnosis may create a dilemma, for an aneurysm may be small and fusiform, raising doubts as to whether it might have bled. In one patient the only evidence of an aneurysm following subarachnoid hæmorrhage was a little irregularity at the carotid bifurcation and no treatment was undertaken, but four years later after a second subarachnoid hæmorrhage the aneurysm was shown to be considerably enlarged. In this patient the carotid artery was ligated and the post-operative angiogram showed considerable improvement (Fig. 8) but had this aneurysm been in a different situation it might have been clipped and the carotid spared in case it was ever necessary to tie the other carotid for a new aneurysm.

When an aneurysm bleeds the least that can happen is an outpouring of blood into the subarachnoid space. If the bleeding is massive this can be fatal, but lesser degrees of hæmorrhage can produce alarmingly deep coma and yet be followed by a degree of recovery that is truly remarkable, if no other damage results from the rupture.

The extent of the initial rise of intracranial pressure and the brain shift that can occur was demonstrated by cases showing total loss of upward gaze, evidence of mid brain compression which persisted for days after the return to full mental lucidity (Johnson and Yates,

a   *b*   *c*

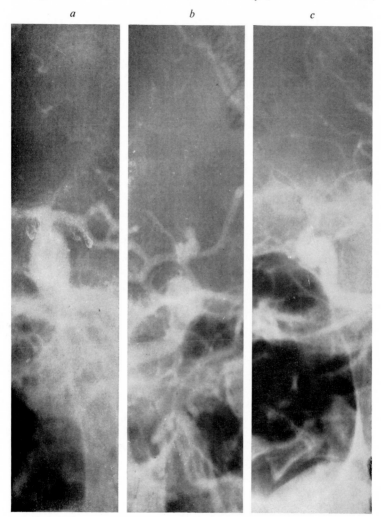

Figure 8. Aneurysm of carotid bifurcation. *a*. initial angiogram; *b*. angiogram 4 years later; *c*. angiogram 5 months after common carotid ligation.

1956). The presence of more than a slight amount of blood in the cerebrospinal fluid will initiate an illness developing over a few days with worsening of the patient's condition and with symptoms and signs akin to meningitis.

If an operation is undertaken in the early phase it may be extremely difficult to locate the point of rupture of an aneurysm. A neighbouring clot may make it certain that a particular aneurysm has leaked, but the lesion on the aneurysm itself may be represented by a clot of a few mm in diameter or there may be no sign at all that the aneurysm has bled, except that the wall is thin and transparent, and there is adjacent clot or yellow staining. (Most illustrations of aneurysms are taken from necropsy studies, which are inevitably the most severe cases and unfortunately tend to convey a more florid appearance than is usually seen at operation.)

Operations may sometimes be more safely performed within a few hours of the first hæmorrhage than at a later date.

The patient who is having repeated subarachnoid leaks of such severity that he loses consciousness and perhaps becomes opisthotonic with each hæmorrhage, and yet recovers completely within an hour or two is helped by improved pre-operative management. Induction of anæsthesia and surgery is hazardous in such cases because of the risk of further hæmorrhage. It is our practice with these patients to lower the blood pressure by means of an Arfonad drip and use an operating table with the head raised. The blood pressure is lowered to 60 mm mercury or until the patient is about to faint, and is kept at this level for about half an hour; a fall below this level can be corrected by levelling the table. I believe that this procedure has been life-saving on a number of occasions, and has enabled operation to be safely carried out within the next few hours. A further consequence of hæmorrhage is the formation around the aneurysm of a dense hard clot that engulfs all the vessels and finally becomes organized. This may make an operation extremely difficult and hazardous, and is one reason why early operation is advantageous.

Another and more troublesome consequence of leakage from an aneurysm is the development of arterial spasm. This may be seen in an angiogram, but has to be distinguished from variations in blood flow and pre-existing narrowing of an artery. The spasm may be so severe that the aneurysm fails to fill. There are various theories as to the cause of spasm—neurogenic, chemical and mechanical, but none is proven. The force of blood discharged from an aneurysm is not inconsiderable and may produce spasm by stretching perforating

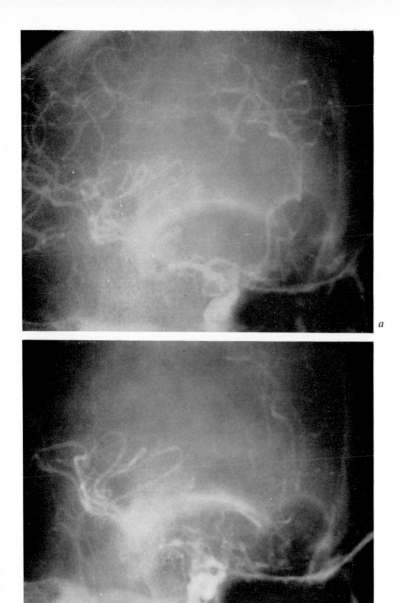

Figure 9a. Angiogram 2 days after subarachnoid hæmorrhage. Small carotid aneurysm—no spasm. *b.* Angiogram 10 days later—severe spasm, no aneurysmal filling.

vessels and arachnoid bands (Dott, 1953). I have been impressed by the kinking and distortion of vessels both when seen at operation and when measured on consecutive angiograms. The distortion would seem to be sufficient to reduce blood flow. The presence of firm blood clot around a narrow vessel may play a part in prolonging the spasm sometimes for weeks, and it is possible too that chemical breakdown products (e.g. serotonin) as well as mechanical factors are important. Yet spasm may occur at any time after the initial hæmorrhage and angiogram (typically within four or five days) and without evidence of further hæmorrhage, as shown by a normal CSF on lumbar puncture (Fig. 9). The use of such preparations as papaverine and Rogitine even when injected into the carotid artery has been disappointing in the treatment of severe arterial spasm. Spasm certainly occurs after operation and may sometimes be severe yet not be associated with any symptoms. The dissection of vessels from dense arachnoidal adhesions may immediately relieve "spasm" of several weeks' duration. The local application to blood vessels of such substances as papaverine has not in my experience been helpful in relieving anything but mild spasm, such as may be induced by manipulation at operation. In two instances I have observed the narrowing of spasm to become permanent; in one, subsequent histological examination suggested that the spasm had induced endothelial hypertrophy, although the increased flow through a narrowed vessel might be expected to militate against effects of hypertrophy.

Spasm may cause distant thromboses, although pathologists are perhaps too ready to assume that spasm has been the causative factor in distal infarctions without evidence of thrombosis or embolism: the initial hæmorrhage may be extremely disruptive and adjoining vessels may be kinked and virtually obliterated perhaps for hours, long enough to cause peripheral ischæmic infarction. Some neurosurgeons (Pool and Potts, 1965) will not operate in the presence of spasm; I have not been so rigid as this, weighing the risks of further hæmorrhage and operating unless there was evidence of gross neurological dysfunction or, equally sinister, progressive deterioration in the patient's conscious state, attributable to the spasm and not to recurrent hæmorrhage or clot. It would seem certain that moderate hypothermia is not helpful in such cases and may, in the presence of spasm, increase the risk to the patient by reducing blood flow. During some of the operations done under deep hypothermia I spent the waiting hour during the re-warming phase observing the exposed brain and its blood vessels. In two cases mechanical tweaking of small arteries failed to produce spasm at 14°C, but produced spasm extremely readily when a temperature of 28°C was reached.

The correlation of the degree and extent of spasm, and the degree of neurological dysfunction is not always as close as might be wished, and spasm cannot be blamed for all "aneurysmal ills". Indeed many patients with all the physical signs suggestive of spasm have completely normal arterial trees. By analogy with the development of hemiplegia following carotid ligation, spasm sufficient to produce ischæmia should occur some time before the onset of the neurological signs, and it could be that the spasm seen on an arteriogram is not at that moment harmful unless the patient is deteriorating progressively. Furthermore, if, as may happen, the neurological signs disappear and the spasm persists, it is abundantly clear that the circulation must be adequate. So the clinical effect of spasm may be the result of an incident at some moment in time and cannot be measured against the blood flow through narrowed vessels seen in the angiogram.

Potter evaluated the reduction in blood flow in our cases of spasm using Poiseuille's Law of fluid flow (Johnson *et al.*, 1958; Johnson and Potter, 1958; Potter, 1959, 1961). Some of his findings were alarming in terms of the reduced flow to the brain. However, a recent view is that blood is a plastic and flows more like a lubricating oil than a simple fluid, and its distribution is probably better understood in terms of these laws. Viscosity and other properties (including the cellular structure) are of great importance, and changing these by the use of such substances as low molecular weight Dextran may have a beneficial effect on the circulation. If the abundance of information relating to arterial spasm in association with intracranial hæmorrhage makes so little contribution to the understanding of its causation, it would certainly seem to me to suggest that it is a very unlikely cause of migraine!

The most severe complications of hæmorrhage from aneurysms include intracerebral and subdural hæmatomas, disturbances of function of the mid brain and of other levels of the brain stem sometimes associated with extensive and fatal secondary hæmorrhages. In some of these cases, of course, spasm is an added complication. Patients with localized blood clots have been treated in the same manner as patients with primary cerebral hæmorrhage (c.f. p. 104) except that when an angioma or an aneurysm has been shown to be present this has been operated upon just as soon as it was deemed safe and possible. It has been my experience that aneurysms of the middle cerebral artery are extremely dangerous in view of their tendency to bleed again at a short interval. However, the evacuation of blood clot from the Sylvian fissure and temporal lobe after leakage from these aneurysms can be far more safely accomplished than the removal of more deeply situated blood clots, which result from hæmorrhage from aneurysms of the anterior cerebral or posterior communicating arteries. Furthermore, aneurysms of the middle cerebral artery can be cured in the acute phase with much less risk of complication, than those arising elsewhere.

The treatment of aneurysms

There are insufficient criteria by which either all patients with aneurysms or any particular grouping of patients with aneurysms as judged by site of the aneurysm, age, blood pressure, interval from initial hæmorrhage, or the number of hæmorrhages, can be unequivocally selected for any particular form of treatment. Field studies such as the cooperative collection of the National Institutes of Health (Sahs, 1965), and the method of arbitrary selection of cases for surgical as opposed to conservative treatment (McKissock and Walsh, 1956) are producing statistics, but because of the wide variation of surgical methods and skills (in fact the only real constant is the group treated conservatively) it is problematical whether these statistics are of sufficient value to deter or encourage the individual surgeon. The greatest knowledge and advances have come from personal series (often small) in which a close study of individual cases has been made, supported by meticulous documentation. I have always believed that one of the surgical skills is case selection, and indeed this should become wider and more comprehensive as knowledge accumulates, and as technical and other skills increase, although such a changing attitude to case selection ruins statistics. I believe that there are certain cases that can be operated upon and cured with a mortality little different from that for appendicectomy, that this can be confidently predicted, and that it would be wrong to deny patients the benefit of this form of treatment. A detailed study of the outstanding problems and experimentation with new techniques, materials and instruments, should bring further patients with aneurysms within the field favourable for treatment. Experience may enable the risk of a further hæmorrhage occurring and the subsequent chance of survival, to be weighed against the risk of operation at different stages. The main difficulty is our inability to predict how a particular aneurysm will behave.

Ligation of the carotid artery in the neck (the common carotid is usually favoured as being slightly safer and only slightly less effective than the internal carotid) was the original form of treatment.

Although it may be considered unscientific in that it reduces the flow of blood to the brain (which may already be damaged), rarely cures the aneurysm and does not always prevent early recurrence of hæmorrhage, yet the low morbidity and the favourable long term results are such that it still remains a yardstick for alternative forms of treatment. It is a very useful form of treatment for any aneurysm that can only be operated upon directly at great risk, and is of special value in the treatment of giant aneurysms of the circle of Willis and of aneurysms of the internal carotid trunk. Carotid ligation may be life saving in cases of repeated hæmorrhage where facilities for elaborate intracranial operations do not exist. A study undertaken before the extension of the field of intracranial surgery showed that of 250 cases of aneurysms (not all of which had bled), 142 patients had their carotids ligated, the mortality being 15 per cent on a long term follow-up (Jefferson, 1951b). In recent years carotid artery ligation has not been used on my unit if the patient was hemiplegic or if the level of consciousness was severely depressed. A study of morbidity after carotid ligation in 1951 showed that 7 per cent of all patients developed post-ligation weakness, but that only 5 per cent remained disabled by hemiplegia. At that time carotid ligation carried out for acute cases of hæmorrhage from aneurysms was associated with a mortality of 50 per cent (Johnson, 1952), or more correctly, 50 per cent of patients recovered and were discharged from hospital after carotid ligation; figures that are certainly now improved by careful selection for direct operation. The morbidity of carotid artery ligation has been reduced to negligible proportions by the thorough examination of the cross circulation angiographically, by avoiding the closure of one carotid if the other is narrowed, or has recently (within 48 hours) been subjected to puncture for angiography, and by the slow closure of the carotid over a period of 2 or 3 days by means of a clamp (Selverstone, 1957). I use a simplified clamp (Dimant, 1959), and when the carotid is fully occluded, ligatures previously passed round the vessel are tied and the clamp is removed. Certain precautions are necessary: the clamp must never be so tightened that it crushes the intima—a slight trickle of blood will not influence the end result and will prevent thrombus formation; the distal ligature must be well clear of the clamp and must be carefully tied before the clamp is in any way disturbed.

The method of direct operation on aneurysms employed by my unit has consisted of careful dissection, depression of the blood pressure by the use of Arfonad often to 50 mm mercury during critical phases of the sac manipulation, and the actual clipping of the neck. During the operation the stretched sac shrinks a little and regains some of its elasticity, occasionally main supplying vessels are temporarily clipped and Scoville's spring clip has proved ideal for this. The aneurysmal neck has been occluded by clips made in various sizes and shapes from silver wire and plate, the jaws being fashioned in a curve so that the tips close first and enclose the aneurysm. After selection for size they can be insinuated round the neck and often under important branches, partially closed and adjusted for position, and then finally closed. For this a straight artery forcep without a ratchet has proved to be the most versatile instrument. If successfully applied and closed these clips have presented no subsequent problems since they were first used in 1951, but spring clips, although at times easy to apply, have on several occasions slipped, and in other instances there have been subsequent slight leakages perhaps due to pressure erosion near the neck of the aneurysm. Other methods have their adherents and there is a whole array of special clips some with locks and special applicators for all situations.

Gallagher (1963, 1964) described an ingenious method of producing thrombosis by pilo-injection, driving hog's bristles into an aneurysmal sac by means of a special air gun, but this method has not proved of very great value in the very aneurysms it would have been most useful, i.e. those that could not be treated any other way. Mullan *et al.* (1964) quoted by Pool and Potts (1965) has introduced an ingenious method of changing the electric charge on the aneurysmal lining by using a stainless steel wire inserted into the aneurysm by stereotaxis, a small current is passed for several hours, and thrombosis induced, but the early evidence is that some of the thromboses have not been permanent. This approach was based on the work of Markovitch (1963) who demonstrated that the normal electro-negative charge of the intima of 5 mv changed to an electro-positive charge of up to 10 mv when it was damaged and it appeared that when this happened thrombosis was likely to occur. Even more ingenious is the injection into the aneurysm itself of carbonyl iron powder in human serum to produce clotting. This is carried out stereotactically, controlled by abutting magnetic probes, but too few cases have been treated for the results to be assessed (Alkne, Fingerhut, and Rand, 1967). Finally, from the time of the earliest operations on aneurysms, attempts have been made to strengthen the sac; muscle, cotton wool, cellophane, fibrin foam, and materials such as nylon and terylene have all been used. However, if the aneurysm can be completely dissected so that it can be totally surrounded by one of these materials it is usually possible to do something more curative, either by clipping or ligature. The other problem is that this wrapping does not prevent recurrent hæmorrhage in the early stages, although it may be excellent in the long term (Fig. 7). The search for a more rigid material that would prevent early hæmorrhage as well as being beneficial in the long term has not as yet produced the ideal answer. Dutton (1956) used acrylic resin, Selverstone and Ronis (1958) used epoxy polyamide but with plastic adhesives so that it would attach itself to the wet aneurysm. These methods are not greatly used because more curative methods are more appealing, but rigidity in the aneurysmal covering would add support even if this covering were not all embracing. This added rigidity might well be a factor in the production of better immediate results than had been obtained with the softer materials. There is no doubt that the foreign proteins in fibrin foam eventually produce the most intense reaction. Although, when placed on an unruptured aneurysm, it may fail to adhere sufficiently to prevent a leakage during the next few days, when held in position over a ruptured sac it has, when involved in the clotting, proved of immediate and lasting value.

The mortality of treating aneurysms is low in favourable cases, but very high for the bad risk cases. Are there any reasons for this discrepancy? One explanation is that many of the poor risk patients are going to die anyway, even in the absence of further hæmorrhage; the damage caused by initial hæmorrhage proves fatal although not immediately. Another reason is that some patients selected for treatment, who die before operation can be undertaken, are included in this category and so produce a further adverse loading. There may be aspects of the operation itself which make a demand on the damaged brain, and which might be circumvented if they were recognized.

A detailed analysis of the operative failures and of the post-operative complications has revealed some of the answers. First of all the anæsthetic: few advances have achieved more for all branches of neurosurgery than those made in this field. Few drugs are without some effect on the brain, and so ideally the very minimum of medication should be employed and unless hypothermic procedures have been used the patient should return immediately to his pre-operation state (or to an improved state if a hæmatoma has been removed) at the end of an operation. Ideally management consists of accurately controlled respiration, with full curarization (the slightest return of muscle tone frequently unrecognizable by the anæsthetist will cause

5

increased bleeding and increased brain turgidity), and the use of Pentobarbitone and very little else.

Hypothermia is used less and less and is only necessary when it is planned to occlude major blood vessels for some time. There is a suggestion that post-operative recovery is smoother when hypothermia is not used. Deep hypothermia has rarely been used and only on occasions when it was considered that moderate hypothermia would not permit a large central aneurysm to be dissected and the entry and leaving vessels preserved in the period of time allowed by temporary vessel occlusion (Fig. 10). There is no doubt that lowering the blood pressure can be damaging, and there is little evidence that mild hypothermia prevents this. Because of this I do as much of the operation as is possible at a normal blood pressure. There are certain anæsthetic drugs and procedures which, in my opinion, can be damaging; the use of opiates, the use of pethidine, the use of haloperidols and phenoperidene; the reduction of blood pressure by the use of halothane, increased intra-thoracic pressure, and finally methods of rapid cooling especially using hypercarbia, which has on a few occasions produced an incredible increase in brain tension.

Important factors at the operation itself are: the most careful retraction of the brain (and in this the planning of an adequate approach is very helpful), great gentleness in handling all the blood vessels so that spasm is not caused or accentuated, the minimum dissection, and especially the avoidance of occlusion of small blood vessels wherever possible.

There is a special risk attached to treatment of aneurysms of the posterior communicating artery; often this artery may be clipped with impunity, but there is grave risk when it is a large vessel, and is, in fact, the posterior cerebral artery arising from the carotid. A large posterior cerebral artery may supply perforating arteries to the basal ganglia and if these thrombose they cause morbidity. This morbidity is greater and the recovery less complete if the patient is already disabled.

Finally there is the risk of hæmorrhage at operation, the risk of aneurysmal rupture, and it is to prevent this that so many of the special procedures have been devised, e.g. the progressive temporary clipping operation (Pool, 1962) in which both carotids are clipped and then both anterior cerebrals, and perhaps the peripheral anterior cerebrals, before the anterior communicating aneurysm is permanently clipped. Elective circulatory arrest for short periods (Small and Stephenson, 1966; Small et al. 1966) and deep hypothermia might assist in the management of such a case.

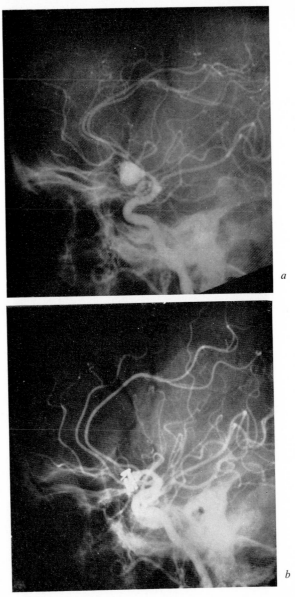

Figure 10*a and b.* Pre-operative (*a*) and post-operative (*b*) angiogram of large anterior communicating aneurysm which was dissected and obliterated under deep hypothermia with total cardiac arrest for 35 minutes; it was considered that it might be necessary to cut off the circulation for rather more time than could be achieved with moderate hypothermia; hæmorrhage into the basal ganglia on the left as the result of anti-coagulation marred an otherwise excellent result.

Moderate hypothermia, although used less and less, has been the means of providing good anæsthetic conditions, and of encouraging many neurosurgeons to operate on difficult aneurysms.

The Arteriovenous Malformations

Arteriovenous malformations may cause fits, headaches, and bruits disturbing to the patient, and may rarely cause raised intracranial pressure. They are a source of hæmorrhage (1 per cent of cerebrovascular accidents (Zimmerman, 1963)), and although they may remain quiescent for almost the whole of the patient's life they have been known to cause severe and fatal hæmorrhage at the age of 60 and over. 42 per cent of Pool's (1962) 48 cases presented with hæmorrhage, and in the Manchester series many of the cases had repeated hæmorrhages over the years, Jefferson (1948). Pool and Potts (1965) collected 523 cases and found that excision gave good results in 74 per cent, had a total morbidity and mortality of 26 per cent against 44 per cent good results and 56 per cent total mortality and morbidity for medical and/or X-ray therapy. There is no doubt that increasing experience has enabled most of the angiomas to be safely excised without gross neurological deficit. This success has been achieved by lowering the blood pressure at intervals during the operation (hypothermia has only been used when it was planned to cut off main vessels for any length of time). The dissection, usually done with a normal blood pressure, is commenced close to the vessels, and sometimes draining veins are used as guides to a deep angioma. Whenever bleeding from small vessels becomes troublesome during the dissection the blood pressure is lowered with Arfonad to 50 mm Hg for as short a period as possible (Fig. 11).

To demonstrate all the feeding vessels angiography must be comprehensive, and serial views are invaluable. Angiomas can be delineated very satisfactorily with radioactive isotopes (Feindel et al., 1961).

Deep X-ray therapy is only used if an angioma is inoperable or if the patient refuses an operation. In a few cases the angioma has been cured, by such treatment, as evidenced by later angiography. It has not been possible to determine the moment of cure, but it may not occur for some two or three years, and therefore would seem to be due to the production of endarteritis in the abnormal vessels by the irradiation. An almost identical angiogram to Fig. 11 is shown in Fig. 12. This angioma was cured by deep X-ray therapy, which was used because the patient refused operation. However, even if only a small number have been cured without adverse consequences, they

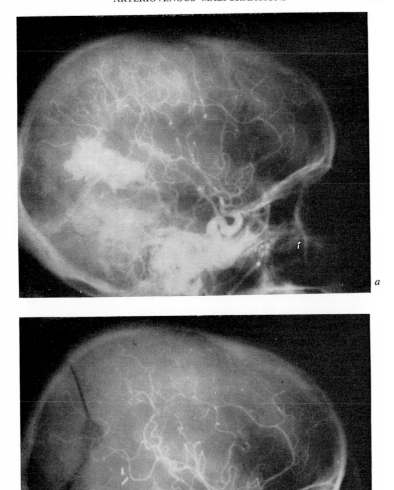

Figure 11*a and b*. Angiomatous malformation, pre-operative (*a*)
and post-operative (*b*) angiograms; total excision.

represent a definite gain, for they have all been patients who for one reason or another could not be treated by surgery.

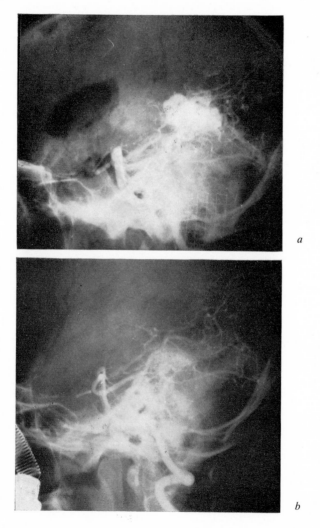

a

b

Figure 12. Similar angioma to Fig. 7. Angiograms prior to X-ray therapy (*a*), and 6 years later (*b*).

Conclusions

Finally, when all known steps have been taken to avoid the production of further damage by operation, and when the benefit of experience has been used in selecting patients for operation, or choosing the time of operation, is there any form of management that will help to reduce morbidity and mortality in patients with cerebral hæmorrhage? Studies of blood electrolytes have failed to reveal any strikingly significant abnormalities (Buckell *et al.*, 1967). Dehydration, of course, can be a problem and should be corrected. Reversal of the normal ratio of plasma proteins may indicate a grave prognosis (Lomax, 1957). Prolonged hypothermia has not proved to be very helpful and can be dangerous; the body temperature should be kept at a normal level and cooling may be necessary to avoid hyperpyrexia. In some patients diuretics have been helpful, and there are occasional reports of patients responding dramatically to corticosteroids. My experience of steroids has been disappointing; I have little evidence that true brain swelling is reduced, nor have I been convinced that any one form of steroid therapy is any better than any other, although of course the effective dose will vary. The use of hypotensive drugs has been advocated in the belief that a small reduction in blood pressure minimized the risk of further hæmorrhage; however, in many of my patients not only has a moderate fall in blood pressure failed to prevent further hæmorrhage, but has on some occasions increased the brain damage. Dissolution of clots by fibrinolysis may prove to be an important factor in recurrent hæmorrhage. Inhibition of fibrinolysis with E. amino caproic acid is now under trial. As yet we have no means of halting the progressive deterioration likened by Jefferson (1951a) to a chain reaction, which occurs in some patients after cerebral hæmorrhage.

References

ALKNE, J. F., FINGERHUT, A., and RAND, R. W. (1967). *J. Neurol. Neurosurg. Psychiat.*, **30**, 159.

BREMER, J. L. (1943). *Arch. Path.*, **35**, 819.

BUCKELL, M., RICHARDSON, A., and SARNER, M. (1967). *J. Neurol. Neurosurg. Psychiat.*, **29**, 291.

CARMICHAEL, R. (1945). *J. Path. Bact.*, **57**, 345.

CHARCOT, J. M., and BOUCHARD, C. (1868). *Arch. Physiol. norm. Path.*, **1**, 110, 643.

COLE, F. M., and YATES, P. O. (1967). *J. Path. Bact.*, **93**, 393.

CRAWFORD, T. (1959). *J. Neurol. Neurosurg. Psychiat.*, **22**, 259.

DIMANT, S. (1959). *Brit. J. Surg.* **46**, 333.

DOTT, N. M. (1953). Contribution to 5th International Neurological Congress, Lisbon. Personal communication.

DUTTON, J. E. M. (1956). *Brit. med. J.*, **2**, 585.
ELLIS, A. G. (1909). *Proc. path. Soc. Philad.*, **12**, 197.
EPPINGER, (1887). *Arch. klin. Chir.*, 35, Supplement 1.
FEINDEL, W., ROVIT R. L. and STEPHENS-NEWSHAM, L. (1961) *J. Neurosurg.*, **18**, 811.
FORBUS, W. D. (1930). *Bull. Johns Hopk. Hosp.*, **47**, 239.
FOX, J. A., and HUGH, A. E. (1966). *Brit. Heart J.*, **28**, 388.
GALLAGHER, J. P. (1963). *J. Amer. med. Ass.*, **183**, 231.
GALLAGHER, J. P. (1964). *J. Neurosurg.*, **21**, 129.
GREEN, F. H. K. (1930). *J. Path. Bact.*, **33**, 71.
HACKEL, H. (1927). *Virchows Arch. path. Anat.*, **266**, 630.
HANBY, W. B. (1952). *Intracranial Aneurysms*, Springfield, Ill., Charles C. Thomas.
HASSLER, O., *Ann. Scient. Mtg., Houston Neurol. Soc.*, March 1964.
HOUSEPIAN, E. M., and POOL, J. L. (1958). *J. Neuropath. exp. Neurol.*, **171**, 409.
JEFFERSON, G. (1948). *Rev. neurol.*, **18**, 6.
JEFFERSON, G. (1951a). *Surg. Gynec. Obstet.*, **93**, 444.
JEFFERSON, G. (1951b). *Proc. roy. Soc. Med.*, **45**, 300.
JOHNSON, R. T. (1952). *Proc. roy. Soc. Med.*, **45**, 301.
JOHNSON, R. T., and YATES, P. O. (1956). *Acta radiol.* (*Stockh.*), **46**, 242.
JOHNSON, R. T., POTTER, J. M., and REID, R. G. (1958). *J. Neurol. Neurosurg. Psychiat.*, **21**, 68.
JOHNSON, R. T., and POTTER, J. M. (1958). *Acta III*. Internationalis Angiologorum Congressus, pps. 299–302.
LOMAX, P., (1957) *Lancet* **i**, 904.
MARKOVITCH, B. (1963). *Cleveland clin. Quart.*, **30**, 241.
McKISSOCK, W., and WALSH, L. (1956). *Brit. med. J.*, **1**, 559.
MULLAN, S., RAIMONDI, A., VAILATI, G., REYS, C., and DOBBEN, G. Annals Meeting Harvey Cushing Society, Los Angeles, April 1964.
PADGET, D. H. (1948). *Contr. Embryol. Carneg. Inst.*, **33**, 205.
POOL, J. L., and POTTS, D. G. (1965). *Aneurysms and Arteriovenous Anomalies of the Brain, Diagnosis and Treatment*. New York, Hoeber.
POOL, J. L. (1962). *J. Neurosurg.*, **19**, 136.
POTTER, J. M. (1959). *Brain*, **82**, 367.
POTTER, J. M. (1961). *Wld. Neurol.*, **2**, 576.
ROSS RUSSELL, R. W. (1963). *Brain*, **86**, 425.
RUSSELL, DOROTHY S. (1954). *Proc. roy. Soc. Med.*, **47**, 689.
SAHS, A. L. (1965). In *Intracranial Aneurysms and Subarachnoid Hæmorrhage*, Ed. W. S. Fields and A. L. Sahs, pp. 486–601. Springfield, Ill., Charles. C. Thomas.
SELVERSTONE, B., and RONIS, N. (1958). *Bull. Tufts-New Eng. med. Cent.*, **4**, 8.
SELVERSTONE, B. (1957) Personal Communication quoted by DIMANT, S. (1959). *Brit J. Surg.*, **46**, 333.
SMALL, J. M., and STEPHENSON, S. C. (1966). *Lancet* **i**. 569
SMALL, J. M., STEPHENSON, S. C., CAMPKIN, T. V., DAVISON, P. H., and McILVEEN, D. J. S. (1966). *Lancet* **i**. 570.
SYMONDS, C. P. (1924). *Quart. J. Med.*, **18**, 25.
SYMONDS, C. P. (1952). *Proc. roy. Soc. Med.*, **45**, 302.
TAYLOR, P. E. (1961). *Neurology*, **2**, 225.
TUTHILL, C. R. (1953). *Arch. Path.*, **16**, 453.
WALKER, A. E., and ALLEGRE, G. W. (1954). *J. Neuropath. exp. Neurol.*, **13**, 248.
ZIMMERMAN, H. M. (1963). *Bull. N.Y. Acad. Med.*, **36**, 263.

CHAPTER 7

MISCELLANEOUS ADVANCES

THE NEUROLOGICAL MANIFESTATIONS OF FOLATE DEFICIENCY

M. C. BRAIN

THE classical neurological picture of subacute combined degeneration, with or without impairment in cerebral function, has long been recognized as being due to deficiency of vitamin B_{12}. Such patients are often not anæmic, but will show macrocytosis of red cells and hypersegmentation of neutrophils in the peripheral blood, and megaloblastic erythropoiesis in bone marrow biopsies. Subacute combined degeneration is associated with levels of serum vitamin B_{12} of less than 80 $\mu\mu$g per ml (normal range 140 to 900 $\mu\mu$g per ml) and values of less than 50 $\mu\mu$g per ml may occur in the absence of anæmia (Mollin, 1959). In contrast the level of serum folate is raised to very high levels in such non-anæmic patients (Waters and Mollin, 1965).

It is becoming increasingly recognized that not all patients who have neurological disease and macrocytic anæmia have a deficiency of vitamin B_{12}. Some of these patients, who rarely have the classical features of subacute combined degeneration, have shown a response to treatment with folate, both in respect of the neurological symptoms and signs, and also of their anæmia. The recognition and treatment of folate deficiency, and its differentiation from deficiency of vitamin B_{12}, has become an increasingly important problem for the neurologist, as many of the commonly employed anticonvulsant drugs, phenobarbitone, phenytoin, and primidone, have been found to be folate antagonists, and are capable of inducing or exacerbating a folate deficiency state, and thus causing a macrocytic anæmia.

Neurological Features

These are not clear cut, and may not be due to deficiency of folate alone. Indeed $4\frac{1}{2}$ months of folate deprivation produced insomnia, forgetfulness and irritability but no objective neurological signs (Herbert, 1962).

Long *et al.* (1963) described the occurrence of megaloblastic anæmia and cutaneous hypalgesia below the knees, with normal vibration and position sense, in a 47-year-old man being treated for epilepsy with phenytoin, phenobarbitone and primidone. Both the anæmia and the sensory loss improved after folate treatment. Anand (1964) described a 64-year-old man receiving the same anticonvulsant drugs with a megaloblastic anæmia, peripheral neuropathy, incontinence and dementia, who showed no response to treatment with vitamin B_{12}, but who made a striking improvement with folate therapy. Grant *et al.* (1965) gave a detailed account of 10 patients with neurological disease and megaloblastic erythropoiesis. Two patients had subacute combined degeneration, and responded to vitamin B_{12}. One patient with features of subacute combined degeneration and a low serum vitamin B_{12} did not respond to treatment with vitamin B_{12}. Seven patients had a low serum folate, but normal serum vitamin B_{12} levels in association with neurological disease. Only one of these patients was anæmic. Four had a paraplegia, with a peripheral neuropathy, but did not improve objectively or subjectively with folate treatment. Three patients with only a peripheral neuropathy—involving both cutaneous and proprioceptive sensibility, without evidence of spinal cord damage, had both subjective and objective improvement after folate treatment. None of the patients described by Grant and her co-authors had been taking anticonvulsant drugs, nor was there evidence that they had a disorder causing malabsorption of folate. It seemed probable that the folate deficiency was of nutritional origin, a suggestion supported by dietary histories. The possible deficiency of other vitamins which may have been responsible for the neurological disease in these patients which was corrected with improvement of the appetite and diet could not be refuted by the authors.

Strachan and Henderson (1967) described two elderly women, aged 69 and 70 years with progressive dementia and macrocytic anæmia with low levels of serum folate and normal levels of vitamin B_{12}. Both the patients showed a progressive improvement in mental function, in EEG records, and in the anæmia following folate treatment. The authors argued convincingly that the improvement in cerebral function was more likely to be due to the correction of the folate deficiency than of the anæmia or to any other factors.

The Ætiology of Folate Deficiency

These accounts suggest that prolonged folate deficiency may cause a disturbance of function of both the peripheral and central nervous system. The occurrence of dementia may be an important factor in the ætiology of the deficiency as such patients show a disinclination to eat and so to take adequate amounts of folate in their diet. Read *et al.* (1965) reported the occurrence of low serum folate levels in the elderly and indicated that this was due to nutritional deficiency, owing to the low folate content of the average diet of these elderly people. In a survey of 100 consecutive admissions to a geriatric hospital Batata *et al.* (1967) found that low serum folate levels were associated with organic brain disease. In these patients it was thought that the low folate level reflected lack of interest in food. The effects of folate treatment were not described, but if deficiency in folate is liable to impair mental function with a progressive reduction in food and folate intake an exacerbation of the deficiency is likely to occur.

The occurrence of neurological disorders in patients with malabsorption of folate has been described by Spencer (1957) and Cooke and Smith (1966). The latter authors were, however, unable to relate the varied neurological disorders they described in patients with idiopathic steatorrhœa to any single factor. Nevertheless it seems probable that abnormalities in the nervous system due to folate deficiency may be encountered in such patients.

Anticonvulsant Drugs and Folate Metabolism

The occurrence of megaloblastic anæmia in patients taking anticonvulsant drugs was described by Mannheimer *et al.* in 1952, and by Badenoch (1964). About 100 cases have been described since. The association has been investigated and discussed in detail by Klipstein (1964) and Reynolds *et al.* (1966). The mechanism of interaction of the drugs phenytoin, primidone, and phenobarbitone, individually or in combination with folate metabolism is incompletely understood. Although low serum folate levels occur in the majority of patients on anticonvulsants, anæmia is rare (Klipstein, 1964; Reynolds *et al.*, 1966). The effect of correction of the folate deficiency on the control of the epilepsy is still uncertain, for although Chanarin *et al.* (1960) described a patient in whom this led to an exacerbation of the epilepsy, Hawkins and Meynell (1958) noted improvement in control of epilepsy in some patients after folate treatment, but owing to the variability in the natural frequency of seizures refrained from drawing conclusions. Yet where, as noted above, mental deterioration has accompanied folate deficiency, improvement in EEG tracings may be associated with folate treatment, and it thus seems likely that the incidence of seizures may be lessened rather than increased, and where folate deficiency becomes apparent it should be corrected.

Diagnosis and Treatment of Folate Deficiency

Deficiency of folate must be suspected in anæmic elderly patients with a history of poor dietary intake, especially when receiving prolonged treatment with barbiturates or other anticonvulsant drugs.

The possibility of folate deficiency is increased by finding a macrocytic anæmia. But the incidence of vitamin B_{12} deficiency is highest in the elderly, and must be distinguished from folate deficiency. This can only be done with certainty by assaying the respective vitamins in the serum (Mollin, 1965). When such assays are not available it is necessary to test for histamine fast-gastric achlorhydria, and to measure the absorption of radioactive vitamin B_{12}. The occurrence of subacute combined degeneration in dietary deficiency of vitamin B_{12} (Badenoch, 1954) and in malabsorption due to ileal disease (Richmond and Davison, 1958) indicates the limited value of indirect tests, as neither of these conditions is associated with gastric achlorhydria, and the absorption of vitamin B_{12} was normal in the former. A distinction between the deficiency of vitamin B_{12} and folate may be obtained by measuring the response of the anæmia to treatment with physiological amounts of the respective vitamins (vitamin B_{12} 2 μg i.m. daily, or folic acid 200 μg daily by mouth). Where it is impractical to carry out these investigations or to await the result of therapeutic responses, it would be advisable to obtain two separate samples of serum for vitamin assay and then to start treatment with vitamin B_{12} 1,000 μg weekly, and add folate (15 mg daily by mouth) if there has been no response. Prolonged treatment with folate should not be given to patients with neurological disorders in whom the serum level or the absorption of vitamin B_{12} is unknown in view of the risk of producing an exacerbation of an underlying vitamin B_{12} deficiency, and a consequent severe deterioration in the neurological disorder, recovery from which may be slow and incomplete despite subsequent treatment with large amounts of vitamin B_{12}.

References

ANAND, M. P. (1964). *Scot. med. J.*, **9**, 388.
BADENOCH, J. (1954). *Proc. roy. Soc. Med.*, **47**, 426.
BATATA, M., SPRAY, G. H., BOLTON, F. G., HIGGINS, G., and WOLLNER, L. (1967). *Brit. med. J.*, **2**, 667.

CHANARIN, I., LAIDLAW, J., LOUGHRIDGE, L. W., and MOLLIN, D. L. (1960). *Brit. med. J.*, **2**, 1099.
COOKE, W. T., and SMITH, W. T. (1966). *Brain*, **89**, 683.
GRANT, H. C., HOFFBRAND, A. V., and WELLS, D. G. (1965). *Lancet*, **2**, 763.
HAWKINS, and MEYNELL (1958). *Quart. J. Med. N.S.*, **27**, 45.
HERBERT, V. (1962). *Trans. Ass. amer. Phys.*, **125**, 307.
KLIPSTEIN, F. A. (1964). *Blood*, **23**, 68.
LONG, M. T., CHILDRESS, R. H., and BOND, W. H. (1963). *Neurology (Minneap.)*, **13**, 697.
MANNHEIMER, E., PAKESCH, F., REIMER, E. F., and VETTER, H. (1952). *Med. Klin.*, **47**, 1397.
MOLLIN, D. L. (1959). *Lect. Sci. Basis. Med.*, **7**, 94.
MOLLIN, D. L. (1965). *Proc. roy. Soc. Med.*, **58**, 725.
READ, A. E., GOUGH, K. R., PARDOE, J. L., and NICHOLAS, A. (1965). *Brit. med. J.*, **2**, 843.
REYNOLDS, E., MILNER, G., MATTHEWS, D., and CHANARIN, I. (1966). *Quart. J. Med. N.S.*, **35**, 521.
RICHMOND, J., and DAVISON, S. (1958). *Quart. J. Med.*, *N.S.*, **27**, 517.
SPENCER, I. (1957). *J. Mt. Sinai Hosp.*, **24**, 331.
STRACHAN, R. W., and HENDERSON, J. Q. (1967). *Quart. J. Med. NS.*, **35**, 189.
WATERS, A. H., and MOLLIN, D. L. (1963). *Brit. J. Hœmat.*, **9**, 319.

SUBACUTE SPONGIFORM ENCEPHALOPATHY

MARCIA WILKINSON

This condition was originally described by Jones and Nevin (1954) in a paper entitled "Rapidly progressive cerebral degeneration (subacute vascular encephalopathy)" and is one of a group of degenerative lesions of the brain and brain stem. The onset is usually subacute generally occurring between the ages of 50 and 70. Clinically it is characterized by progressive mental deterioration, focal disturbances and myoclonic epilepsy.

Nevin (1967) considers that whatever its nature, the pathological process in subacute spongiform encephalopathy affects first the grey matter of the cerebral cortex, especially the occipital cortex, and the granular layer of the cerebellum. It then affects the thalamus and basal ganglia and lastly the white matter of the centrum ovale. The large nerve cells are the least affected.

The pathological changes are distinctive and consist of widespread loss of nerve cells in all layers of the cerebral cortex more especially in the occipital lobes with an associated astroglial reaction. There is a varying amount of status spongiosus and electron microscopy shows vesicle formation in the glia and nerve cells.

Nevin (1967) analyzed the clinical features of subacute spongiform encephalopathy basing his study on 60 cases gathered from the literature or studied personally. He found no record of familial incidence, and the age of incidence varied from 31 to 72 years, the most being between 55 and 60. The average duration was 5·3 months.

Clinically it is a progressive disease which is always fatal and occurs in three phases which vary in duration corresponding to the total duration of the disease. The first phase is characterized principally by commencing dementia or a wide variety of focal symptoms indicating lesions in different parts of the brain and cerebellum. In the second phase the focal symptoms tend to be lost in a picture of steadily advancing mental dissolution or organic cerebral confusion very often with wide-spread myoclonus and increasing muscular rigidity. In the third phase there is deepening stupor with increase in the rigidity of the limbs which persists up to a few days before death.

The electroencephalogram is always abnormal, the pattern of abnormality varying with the phase of the disease. In the first phase there is a build-up of slow potentials with diminution of the normal rhythms which may be more marked anteriorly or posteriorly or in one hemisphere or part of a hemisphere corresponding with the initial symptoms of the disease. The second phase is characterized by repetitive sharp wave complexes in intermittent runs or continuously and these again can for a time predominate in one hemisphere. In the third phase there is a lessening in amplitude and there may be only brief bursts of slow and slowed sharp wave activity occurring at long intervals shortly before death. Air studies are usually normal in the early phases of the disease but in patients surviving for a longer time ventricular enlargement and cortical atrophy of a severe degree occur.

References

JONES, D. P., and NEVIN, S. (1954). *J. Neurol. Neurosurg. Psychiat.*, **7**, 148.
NEVIN, S. (1967). *Proc. roy. Soc. Med.*, **60**, 517.

ENCEPHALITIS DUE TO HERPES SIMPLEX

The herpex simplex virus is very widely distributed throughout the world up to 90 per cent of adults possessing antibodies against this agent. Cold sores represent the commonest clinical manifestation of infection with the virus, whereas involvement of the central nervous system is a rare event. It was only in 1941 that the herpes simplex virus was first isolated from human brain after a fatal encephalitic illness. Since that time more than 100 cases of acute necrotizing encephalitis have been recorded and in about three-quarters of them intranuclear inclusions of Cowdry type A have been found. Viral pathogenesis may be confirmed by brain biopsy or by identification of the virus in the fæces or cerebrospinal fluid. It is now generally assumed that the herpes simplex virus is the cause of acute necrotizing encephalitis and this is supported by electron microscopy.

Clinically the picture is of confusion and hyperpyrexia developing over 2–4 days with hemiplegia, neck stiffness and convulsive seizures. Very often the most striking feature is involvement of the temporal lobes and this may cause difficulties in diagnosis, since the clinical picture often suggests a tumour or more especially a brain abscess. The cerebrospinal fluid contains an increased number of white cells up to 1,000 per cu mm with a protein of up to 360 mgs per cent, and sometimes it is heavily blood-stained. Van Bogaert et al. (1955) drew attention to the characteristic asymmetrical lesions, the most striking feature being the involvement of the temporal lobes with softening and numerous hæmorrhagic foci. Microscopically the features of a viral encephalitis are found with, in addition, extensive cell necrosis and neuronophagia. Cowdry type A inclusion bodies are usually found.

Diagnosis of the condition depends on the isolation of the virus from the brain or cerebrospinal fluid, or the demonstration of a rising titre of antibody in the serum. Leider et al. (1965) described 18 patients in whom a laboratory diagnosis of infection due to herpes simplex was made and they considered that a fourfold, or greater, rise in the antibody titre may be accepted as evidence of primary infection with the herpes virus. Acute necrotizing encephalitis carries a very high mortality. Adams and Jennett (1967) described a series of 7 patients 5 of whom died within 14 days of onset of the illness, 1 patient lived for 2 months and the other survived. Some authors have reported good results from the use of ACTH and recently Idoxuridine has been tried. This drug is thought to act by inhibiting viral DNA—polymerase or by becoming incorporated into viral DNA. It is however toxic and has produced leucopenia, stomatitis and alopecia. Three cases have recently been reported where Idoxuridine has been given intravenously in herpes encephalitis and the patients have survived. (Evans et al. 1967, Breeden et al. 1966 and Marshall 1967). It is however such a toxic substance that further trials must be made.

References

ADAMS, J. H., and JENNETT, W. B. (1967). *J. Neurol. Neurosurg. Psychiat.*, **30**, 248.
BREEDEN, C. J., HALL, T. C., and TYLER, H. R. (1966). *Ann. intern. Med.*, **65**, 1050.
EVANS, A. J., GRAY, O. P., MILLER, M. H., VERRIER JONES, E. R., WEEKS, R. D., and WELLS, C. E. G. (1967). *Brit. med. J.*, **2**, 407.
LEIDER, W., MAGOFFIN, R. L., LENNETTE, E. H., and LEONARDS, L. N. R. (1965). *New Engl. J. Med.*, **273**, 341.
MARSHALL, W. J. S. (1967). *Lancet*, **2**, 579.
VAN BOGAERT, L., RADERMECKER, J., and DEVOS, J. (1955). *Rev. neurol.*, **92**, 329.

ENCEPHALITIS DUE TO INFECTION WITH TOXOCARA CANIS

Toxocara canis is a widespread infection of dogs and Woodruff, Thacker and Shah (1964) have shown that 20·7 per cent of all dogs examined in the Home Counties are infected with this parasite.

Any tissue of the body may be invaded by the larvæ and widespread lesions including those in the central nervous system have been described (Dent *et al.*, 1956). The common symptoms are malaise, irritability, anorexia with fever, leucocytosis with a varying degree of eosinophilia, and increase of blood-globulin, especially gamma-globulin (Perlingiero and Gyorgy, 1947). Skin rashes, hepatomegaly which may be associated with jaundice (Karpinski *et al.*, 1956) and respiratory symptoms are common. Less common symptoms are splenomegaly, lymphadenopathy and cardiomegaly.

Neurological Symptoms

Generalized convulsions have been reported in children infected with Toxocara canis (Zuelzer and Apt, 1949; Milburn and Ernst, 1953; Dickson and Woodcock, 1959) but in these cases invasion of the central nervous system by the larvæ was not proved. A fatal case of toxocaral encephalitis in the Netherlands has been recorded (van Thiel, 1960). This was a case of a 19-month old child who died of unrelated serum hepatitis and who was found at necropsy to have microscopic granulomatous lesions with and without larvæ in the spinal cord, pons, cerebellar peduncles and cortex and in the interstices of the leptomeninges. Widespread visceral lesions of identical character were also found. More recently Brain and Allan (1964) have reported a case of encephalitis due to infection with Toxocara canis. Their patient, a woman of 32 originally complained of fits often starting with numbness and tingling in the right lower limb and spreading up the right side and involving the right lips and tongue. Ten months later she developed an illness with fever, headache, generalized aches and pains, nausea, vomiting and abdominal pains, but no diarrhœa. About this time she noticed firm subcutaneous nodules in the right loin and lower extremity. She was found to have a slight right hemiparesis and hemihypæsthesia. No subcutaneous lesions were visible or palpable at that time. Laboratory investigations showed an eosinophil count of 5 per cent in 7,000 white blood cells, hyperglobulinæmia (especially of the gamma-globulin fraction) and the cerebrospinal fluid contained 124 white cells and 55 mg of protein. Occasional eosinophils were found in the CSF and there was an abnormal Lange curve. Electroencephalography showed findings consistent with a focal abnormality in the left parieto-occipital region. All X-ray films were within normal limits and repeated examinations revealed no ova or parasites in the stools. During the time she was under observation two subcutaneous lesions appeared which had the appearance of a granuloma and contained lymphocytes, fibroblasts, plasma cells and eosinophils, the last in large numbers, and areas of necrosis. The toxocaral complement-fixation test was found to be negative but a toxocaral skin test was positive. Brain and Allan treated the patient with diethylcarbamazine (Banocide), 3 mg/kg bodyweight, three times a day for twenty-one days and also gave anticonvulsants. With this treatment the patient's condition improved considerably and the number of fits was reduced. Brain and Allan followed the patient over the next few years and during this time the improvement continued and although she had still got numbness of the right arm, the headaches and fits were not so severe as previously. The authors considered that though toxocaral infection could not be diagnosed with certainty as larval forms were never found, the evidence was strongly in favour of the diagnosis as the positive skin tests appeared reasonably specific. They also point out that toxocaral infection should be considered in all cases of subacute or chronic encephalomyelitis for which no other cause is found, especially if there is eosinophilia in the blood or eosinophils in the cerebrospinal fluid. In such cases the skin test should be carried out. Since larvæ in the central nervous system may not produce symptoms or signs it is wise to investigate the cerebrospinal fluid in all children who are known to be infected by Toxocara. Since the helminth is common to both dogs and cats in this country it should be borne in mind as a possible cause of unexplained epilepsy in childhood. The syndrome is probably commoner than is supposed since the parasite is widespread and few dogs escape infection. Although in most cases the disease is benign and self-limiting it needs to be recognized so that unnecessary investigations can be avoided and the appropriate treatment given.

References

BRAIN, and ALLEN, B. (1964). *Lancet*, **1**, 1355.

DENT, J. H., NICHOLS, R. L., BEAVER, P. C., CARRERA, G. M., and STAGGERS, R. J. (1956). *Amer. J. Path.*, **32**, 777.

DICKSON, W., and WOODCOCK, R. C. (1959). *Arch. Dis. Childh.*, **34**, 63.

KARPINSKI, F., EVERTS-SUAREZ, E., and SAWIZ, W. (1956). *Amer. J. Dis. Child.*, **92**, 34.

MILBURN, C. L., and ERNST, K. F. (1953). *Pediatrics*, **11**, 358.

PERLINGIERO, J. G., and GYORGY, P. (1947). *Amer. J. Dis. Child.*, **73**, 34.

VAN THIEL, P. (1960). *Ned. T. Geneesk.*, **104**, 1104.

WOODRUFF, A. W., THACKER, C. K., and SHAH, A. I. (1964). *Brit. med. J.*, **1**, 1001.

ZUELZER, W., and APT, L. (1949). *Amer. J. Dis. Child.*, **78**, 1953.

LEBER'S OPTIC ATROPHY

In Leber's optic atrophy there is characteristically sudden onset of bilateral visual impairment the fields of vision showing central scotomas. Papillitis may be present in the acute stage but later the discs become atrophic. Until recently this was considered to be a rare hereditary disease which was transmitted as a sex-link recessive. Recently Wilson (1963) has put forward the view that Leber's hereditary optic atrophy is essentially a metabolic disorder with varied neurological manifestations.

Symptomatology. The most common symptoms are visual failure, spasticity, hyperreflexia and impairment of posterior column sensation often with burning pain in the back and lower limbs. Ataxia of both cerebellar and sensory type may also occur but except when extrapyramidal signs are prominent, disturbances of tone and co-ordination are usually attributed to motor neurone and/or cerebellar involvement. Adams, Blackwood and Wilson (1966) emphasize the diffuse involvement of the central nervous system which can occur and suggest that these manifestations are not as rare as might have been supposed and that the visual failure which has hitherto been considered as an invariable part of the syndrome does not always occur and that this may give rise to diagnostic difficulties in the sporadic case of diffuse neurological disease without optic atrophy. However in most families in whom Leber's disease occurs, evidence of retrobulbar neuritis or optic atrophy in one or more relatives sooner or later emerges.

Pathology. The changes in the optic nerves characteristically include a total loss of myelin centrally but in addition there may be widespread damage to the central nervous system. Few, if any, parts of the brain or the cord escape and these changes are consistent with the protean clinical manifestations and the progressive course. Adams, Blackwood and Wilson consider that these changes are consistent with a metabolic or toxic ætiology and that there is no pathological evidence to support the suggestion that neurological complications in Leber's disease present a primary demyelinating disorder or that they represent familial multiple sclerosis.

Aetiology. Wilson (1965) has suggested that a failure to detoxicate cyanide to thiocyanate may be the primary defect, and this would explain the association between smoking and Leber's optic atrophy as tobacco smoking is probably the commonest source of significant amounts of cyanide to which patients in most sophisticated communities are exposed. Other sources of cyanide which may be of importance are those arising from infections (Smith, 1964). Studies on cyanide and thiocyanate concentrations in body fluids showed that concentrations of cyanide five times greater than those normally found in sterile samples were found in urine samples contaminated with E. coli. Adams, Blackwood and Wilson therefore suggest that infections with Ps. pyocyaneus and E. coli, particularly in the urinary tract, may be a contributory factor in Leber's disease and might well account for some of the cases occurring in non-smokers. In two of their patients major neurological deterioration probably occurred after the development of urinary tract infection and they had encountered several patients in whom visual deterioration was preceded by infection.

Treatment. If the hypothesis that there is an inability to metabolize cyanide normally is true there are two important approaches to rational prophylaxis and treatment in susceptable families. Firstly, cyanide exposure must be restricted; heavy cigarette smoking is inadvisable and pipe and cigar smoking are probably best avoided altogether, while infections, particularly urinary infections, should be vigorously eradicated. Secondly, in cases where there is actual neurological and ophthalmological damage occurring massive doses of hydroxycobalamin may be of value both for the cyanide-binding ability of this vitamin and for its role in 1-Carbon metabolism. Other therapeutic agents worth considering are those used in acute cyanide poisoning such as sodium thiosulphate and cobalt compounds.

References

ADAMS, J. H., BLACKWOOD, W., and WILSON, J. (1966). *Brain*, **89**, 15.
SMITH, A. D. M. (1964). *Lancet*, **2**, 668.
WILSON, J. (1963). *Brain*, **86**, 347.
WILSON, J. (1965). *Clin. Sci.*, **29**, 505.

WILSON'S DISEASE (HEPATO-LENTICULAR DEGENERATION)

Wilson's disease is a progressive disease of early life which is frequently familial and is characterized by a disorder of copper metabolism leading to degeneration of certain regions of the brain, especially the corpus striatum, cirrhosis of the liver, and clinically by increasing muscular rigidity and tremor. The pathological changes in the nervous system consist of degeneration of ganglion cells with neuroglial overgrowth but without evidence of inflammation or vascular abnormality, the changes being most marked in the putamen. The caudate nucleus is usually similarly affected although to a lesser extent but the globus pallidus is less frequently involved. Similar alterations are often present in other parts of the nervous system, for example in the cerebral cortex, the optic thalamus, the red nucleus and the cerebellum. Macroscopically the most conspicuous abnormality is found in the lenticular nucleus. In about half the recorded cases visible softening and cavitation of both lenticular nuclei have been observed; in other cases the nucleus has appeared shrunken but occasionally its naked eye appearance is normal. In the liver the changes are those of a multilobular cirrhosis and there is often enlargement of the spleen.

Symptoms. Tremor is usually the first symptom and may occur when the limbs are apparently at rest and is increased by voluntary movement. Rigidity soon develops and is present in all cases, resembling in distribution and general character the rigidity of Parkinsonism. Later the limbs become fixed, usually in a position of flexion, and contractions ultimately develop. Voluntary movement is impaired and articulation and deglutition are early and severely affected. Speech may become unintelligible and the patient may even lose entirely the power of articulation. Loss of emotional control is usually present, voluntary laughing and crying may occur and the patient presents a Parkinsonian appearance. There seems also to be some degree of mental deterioration amounting to a mild dementia. Corneal pigmentation may be found (the Kayser-Fleischer Ring): this consists of a zone of golden-brown granular pigmentation about

2 mm in diameter on the posterior surface of the cornea towards the limbus and may be present before any nervous symptoms have developed. The symptoms of cirrhosis of the liver may be inconspicuous but in more than one case they have proved fatal before the patient developed any nervous symptoms.

Most patients have a low serum copper (normal 86–112 μg per cent) a low cæruloplasmin in the blood (normal 27–38 mg per cent) and a high urinary copper (normal 24-hour excretion 0–26 μg). Both total and α-amino acids are increased in the urine.

Treatment. The precise abnormality causing Wilson's disease is not yet known but the principal manifestations result from tissue damage, mainly in the brain and liver, and the outstanding finding in these sites is excessive deposition of copper. Treatment of Wilson's disease has therefore been directed towards removal of excess copper from the body. Cumings (1948) was the first to suggest treatment for hepato-lenticular degeneration with the chelating agent dimercaprol (BAL) for the removal of copper from the tissues. Other chelating substances such as intravenous aminoacids (Cartwright et al., 1954; Cumings, 1959) have been used and each has been shown to enhance the excretion of copper in the urine. Clinically BAL has been the most effective but it has the disadvantage that it has to be given by intramuscular injection and may be painful. In 1956 Walshe introduced a new chelating agent penicillamine (ββ-dimethyl cysteine) a metabolite of penicillin and this constituted a major therapeutic advance as not only could it be given by mouth but it was a much more effective cpruretic agent than dimercaprol. He found that oral administration of penicillamine to patients with Wilson's disease caused a ten to twenty-fold rise in the renal clearance of copper. In vitro studies suggested that this was achieved by mobilizing copper from cæruloplasmin and making it available for glomerular filtration (Walshe, 1961).

Richmond et al. (1964) have recently discussed in detail three patients who had prolonged and continuous treatment with penicillamine. These patients received continuous penicillamine therapy for five years, four years and four years respectively. They found that penicillamine had a pronounced cpruretic effect in each patient and that this effect was superior to that of dimercaprol or calcium disodium versenate in the one patient in whom comparative studies were made. Another patient showed weight gain and transiently an unusual intracutaneous œdema while receiving the drug; these changes might have been a side effect of penicillamine but apart from diarrhœa at high dose levels at the onset of treatment there was no other evidence of toxicity or intolerance during the long period of administration in the patients studied. They found that there was a delay of several weeks after the institution of penicillamine therapy before clinical improvement occurred. In each patient the response was remarkable, two patients were freed of all disability, Kayser-Fleischer rings being the only clinical stigmata that remained. They found that there was a diminishing cupruretic effect after several months' treatment with penicillamine and they believe this was due to "decoppering" of the patient rather than to the development of a drug resistance. They found that in one patient 0·6 gramme of penicillamine daily was as effective as 1·5 grammes daily and they suggest that in view of the cost of treatment the optimal dose for maintenance therapy should be worked out for each patient.

References

CARTWRIGHT, G. E., HODGES, R. E., GUBLER, C. J., MAHONEY, J. P., DAUM, K., WINTROBE, M. M., and BEAN, W. B. (1954). *J. clin. Invest.*, **33**, 1487.

CUMINGS, J. N. (1948). *Brain*, **71**, 410.

CUMINGS, J. N. (1959). *Proc. roy. Soc. Med.*, **52**, 62.

RICHMOND, J., ROSENOER, V. M., TOMPSETT, S. L., DRAPER, I., and SIMPSON, J. A. (1964). *Brain*, **87**, 619.

WALSHE J. M. (1956). Lancet **1**, 25.

WALSHE, J. M. (1956). *Amer. J. Med.*, **21**, 487.

WALSHE, J. M. (1961). In *Wilson's Disease*, ed. Walshe, J. M. and Cumings, J. N. Oxford.

THE NEUROLOGICAL COMPLICATIONS OF WEGENER'S GRANULOMATOSIS

The earlier writers on the syndrome now known as Wegener's granulomatosis (Klinger, 1931; Rössle, 1933 and Wegener, 1937, 1939) described the characteristic triad of granulomata in the respiratory tract, widespread arteritis and nephritis but made no mention of involvement of the nervous system. Walton (1958) analyzed the clinical features of 56 cases reported in the literature and found that 16 patients (28·6 per cent) showed some evidence of peripheral neuropathy. Drachman (1963) reviewed 104 reported cases and found that more than 50 per cent showed some involvement of the nervous system the largest group (28 per cent) presenting features of a peripheral neuropathy similar to that described in polyarteritis nodosa.

The pathological criteria for the diagnosis of Wegener's granulomatosis as put forward by Godman and Churg (1954) include the following lesions:

1. Granulomata in the respiratory tract.

2. Generalized focal necrotizing vasculitis involving both arteries and veins.

3. Necrotizing and proliferative renal glomerulitis. Other features commonly found are massive necrosis of the spleen and disseminated visceral granulomata.

The neurological manifestations of Wegener's granulomatosis are many and may be either central and/or peripheral in origin. Drachman (1963) divided them into three groups:

1. Continuous invasion of nervous structures by nasal and paranasal granulomata.

2. Involvement by granulomata remote from the respiratory tract.

3. Vasculitis involving the nervous system.

Stern, Hoffbrand and Urich (1965) studied four cases of Wegener's granulomatosis in detail. They found that involvement of the central nervous system was minimal both clinically and pathologically. In the peripheral nervous system the clinical picture was that of "mononeuritis multiplex" of a variable degree of severity. The onset of symptoms was usually sudden with involvement of one or more peripheral nerves. This was followed in rapid succession by further episodes of numbness, paræsthesiæ and weakness in various parts of the limbs until the picture became that of a widespread peripheral neuropathy, both motor and sensory, involving all four limbs particularly their distal parts. All sensory modalities were affected and the tendon jerks were progressively lost during the course of the disease. They found that the pathology of the peripheral nerves resembled closely that described in polyarteritis nodosa with individual variations depending largely on the stage of the disease. Where the involvement of the nervous system was of recent onset arteritic lesions of the vasa nervorum were abundant and, with a few exceptions, in the acute, necrotizing and exudative stages. The affected nerves showed few, if any, degenerative changes and no denervation atrophy was seen in the appropriate muscles. With a neuropathy of longer duration fewer arteries were involved and most of them showed healing or scarred obliterative lesions. The nerves showed advanced Wallerian degeneration of individual bundles. Several motor nerve cells in the anterior horns of the spinal cord showed evidence of axonal reaction, and neurogenic atrophy of variable extent and in different stages of evolution was present in skeletal muscles. These showed a variety of lesions both focal, secondary to vascular occlusion, and diffuse ranging from disuse atrophy to a severe necrotizing myopathy. Active arteritic lesions were commonly seen in the muscle sections and ischæmic damage to the muscle accompanied only a minority of the arterial lesions. Typical infarcts consisted of well circumscribed areas of total fibre necrosis usually with regenerating fibres present at the periphery. Other lesions followed a pattern of partial infarction with scattered foci of necrosis of individual muscle fibres. Similar necrotic lesions had been described in muscle biopsies by Read and Treid (1957) and by Drachman (1963).

The clinical and pathological findings in the peripheral nervous and muscular systems in Wegener's granulomatosis are indistinguishable from those seen in polyarteritis nodosa. There are, however, clinical and pathological reasons for considering Wegener's disease as a separate entity. Early involvement of the respiratory tract is a constant feature and the presenting symptoms are usually facial pain and nasal discharge or less commonly cough, hæmoptysis and dyspnœa. The subsequent clinical course is more rapidly fatal than in polyarteritis nodosa and is usually unaffected by treatment with steroids. The authors are unable to throw much light on the ætiology or pathogenesis of Wegener's granulomatosis but by analogy with polyarteritis nodosa it is thought it might be due to a delayed hypersensitivity reaction. It seems probable that except for occasional involvement of single nerves by spreading granulomata the peripheral neuropathy is ischæmic in nature and secondary to an arteritis of the vasa nervorum. The lesions in the muscles are much more complex in their mechanism, denervation, disuse, ischæmia and probably steroid therapy all playing a part. There is no evidence to suggest that either nerves or muscles in this disease are damaged directly by an antigen-antibody reaction.

References

DRACHMAN, D. A. (1963). *Arch. Neurol. Chic.*, **8**, 145.
GODMAN, G. C., and CHURG, J. (1954). *Arch. Path.*, **58**, 533.
KLINGER, H. (1931). *Frankfurt Z. Path.*, **42**, 455.
READ, A. E., and TREIP, C. S. (1957). *Postgrad. med. J.*, **33**, 199.
RÖSSLE, R. (1933). *Virchows Arch.*, **288**, 780.
STERN, G. M., HOFFBRAND, A. V., and URICH, H. (1965). *Brain*, **88**, 151.
WALTON, E. W. (1958). *Brit. med. J.*, **2**, 265.
WEGENER, F. (1937). *Verh. dtsch. path. Ges.*, **29**, 202.
WEGENER, F. (1939). *Beitr. path. Anat.*, **102**, 36.

REFSUM'S DISEASE

Refsum in 1945 described a condition which he originally called "heredo-ataxia hemeralopia polyneuritiformis" and later referred to as "heredopathia atactica polyneuritiformis" (Refsum, 1946). This is a rare disorder probably inherited as an autosomal Mendelian recessive. The main clinical features of this syndrome are atypical retinitis pigmentosa, cerebellar ataxia and a severe peripheral neuropathy with an increase in the protein in the cerebrospinal fluid. Other abnormalities are often found and these include pupillary abnormalities, nerve deafness, cataracts, bony abnormalities, congenital ichthyosis and cardiomyopathy. The peripheral neuritis runs a varied and unpredictable course. It may remain stationary for a long time or may be progressive but the usual course is one of remissions and relapses. Recently Nevin, Cumings and McKeown (1967) reported the case of a patient who died ten days post-partum following a rapid acute polyneuritic illness.

Refsum (1946) suggested that on clinical grounds this condition might be related to the lipoidoses. Cammermeyer (1956) postulated that the basic defect was an inherited anomaly which influenced the biochemical or biophysical properties of myelin in such a way as to disrupt the protein and lipid layers of the myelin sheath. Recently evidence has accumulated which suggests that a specific disturbance of lipid metabolism exists in Refsum's syndrome. Richterich, Kahlke and others (1963, 1964, 1965) have found storage of a fatty acid, phytanic acid (3, 7, 11, 15-tetramethyl hexadecanoic acid) in the liver, kidney, urine and skeletal muscle of patients with Refsum's disease and Kahlke demonstrated this substance in the serum of 9 patients. Alexander (1966) found high levels of phytanic acid in the brain, sciatic nerve, liver, kidney and heart muscle in one of his patients who came to post-mortem, and Nevin et al. (1967) found abnormal accumulation of phytanic acid in the sera of two of their patients.

Phytanic acid has been synthesized by Steinberg, Avigan, Mize and Baxter (1966) from phytol which is a major constituent of the chlorophyll molecule, and it has been found that phytanic acid accumulates in the liver and plasma of rats fed on phytol. In normal animals phytol and its metabolic products are readily oxidized to CO_2 and appreciable storage in normal rats occurred only when the level of phytol in the diet was high. These experimental results suggest that Refsum's syndrome may be due to a hereditary metabolic defect, possibly enzymatic, which leads to failure to break down phytanic acid synthesized from phytol and that the accumulated phytanic acid is incorporated into the developing myelin sheath. The myelin so formed is less stable than normal and in the peripheral nerves leads to gradual loss of the myelin sheath and to a process of perineural fibrosis.

Nevin *et al.* (1967) consider that with the present evidence it is difficult to know whether the condition is due to the storage of abnormal fatty acids or whether it is the result of some specific disturbance in the degradation of fatty acids. It seems probable, however, that some of the features of Refsum's disease are due to a recessively inherited disorder of lipid metabolism possibly due to a single enzyme defect. Recently Steinberg *et al.* (1967) found that the phytanic acid accumulating in Refsum's disease is primarily of exogenous origin and that the inherited metabolic defect lies in the catabolic pathway. Eldjarn *et al.* (1966) have tried the effect of a diet devoid, as far as possible, of phytanic acid in two patients and found a fall of phytanic acid in the serum and in one case some clinical improvement.

References

ALEXANDER, W. S. (1966). *J. Neurol. Neurosurg. Psychiat.*, **29**, 412.

CAMMERMEYER, J. (1956). *J. Neuropath. exp. Neurol.*, **15**, 340.

ELDJARN, L., TRY, K., STOKKE, O., MUNTHE-KAAS, A. W., REFSUM, S., STEINBERG, D., AVIGAN, J., and MIZE, C. (1966). *Lancet*, **1**, 691.

KAHLKE, W. (1964). *Klin. Wschr.*, **42**, 1011.

KAHLKE, W., and RICHTERICH, R. (1965). *Amer. J. Med.*, **39**, 237.

KLENK, E., and KAHLKE, W. (1963). *Hoppe-Seylers Z. Physiol. Chem.*, **333**, 133.

NEVIN, N. C., CUMINGS, J. N., and MCKEOWN, F. (1967). *Brain*, **90**, 419.

REFSUM, S. (1945) *Nord. Med.*, **28**, 2682.

REFSUM, S. (1946). *Acta psychiat. neurol. scand.*, Suppl., **38**, 1.

RICHTERICH, R., KAHLKE, W., VAN MECHELEN, P., and ROSSI, E. (1963). *Klin. Wsch.*, **41**, 800.

RICHTERICH, R., VAN MECHELEN, P., and ROSSI, E. (1965). *Amer. J. Med.*, **39**, 230.

STEINBERG, D., AVIGAN, J., MIZE, C. E., and BAXTER, J. (1966). *Biochem. biophys. Res. Commun.* (in press).

STEINBERG, D., MIZE, C. E., AVIGAN, J., FALES, H. M., ELDJARN, L., TRY, K., STOKKE, O. J. and REFSUM, S. (1967). *J. clin. Invest.*, **46**, 313.

CHAPTER 8

STEREOTAXIC SURGERY

JOHN HANKINSON

IT IS now twenty years since the first human stereotaxic instrument was described by Spiegel, Wycis, Marks and Lee (1947). This was the first of many adaptations of the original animal stereotaxic instrument devised by R. H. Clarke and used by him and Sir Victor Horsley, as recorded in their paper of 1908. During the past ten years a great number of stereotaxic operations have been performed throughout the world—over 25,000 according to a recent survey by E. A. Spiegel (1965). It seems appropriate, therefore, to attempt an assessment of the contributions and limitations of this type of surgery, to mention some points of technique which are generally accepted and to consider those still causing disagreement.

The stereotaxic method of intracerebral localization depends upon two contrasting disciplines. On the one hand there is an enormously detailed mass of general information on the anatomical mensuration of the human brain and its variations (Spiegel and Wycis, 1952; Talairach et al., 1957; Schaltenbrand and Bailey, 1959; Delmas and Pertuiset, 1959; Van Buren and Maccubbin, 1962). The data derived from this source are then applied to the particular patient, with estimations of individual variability, from radiologically identified reference points chosen by virtue of their proximity to the target area. Thus despite every endeavour biological variation permits a degree of accuracy by anatomical and radiological methods which is still something less than acceptable. On the other hand the mechanical and radiological engineering now available for stereo-taxis is more than adequate and well within the limits imposed by anatomical variability.

TECHNICAL CONSIDERATIONS

Recent published work and conferences devoted to stereotaxic surgery have expressed this by an increasing emphasis on physiological observations during stereotaxic operations as an essential confirmation of localization of a probe or electrode before a permanent lesion is inflicted. A number of techniques have been developed for this purpose. These are either specialized neurophysiological manœuvres such as stimulation or recording techniques or they consist of partial or reversible lesion-making. As might be expected, the results of this type of "experimentation" often defy interpretation, although in practice their immediate purpose, i.e. localization, is usually achieved (Hankinson, 1960). Because of the variety and the often unorthodox nature of the methods employed this difficulty applies particularly to stimulation. Both suppression and augmentation of tremor are reported by different workers who have stimulated the same nucleus with uni-polar or bi-polar electrodes, with currents of different strength and frequency of impulse. Similarly a variety of effects is produced by spread of current to neighbouring structures which may be explicable in terms of localization to a particular operator in the light of his experience but can have little valid application beyond this.

Recording, demanding more sophisticated instrumentation, leads to more consistent and comparable results, but except for the recognition of interfaces between grey and white matter is as yet too refined and too expensive for general use in simple localization. Albe-Fessard *et al.* (1962) and Jasper and Bertrand (1965) have reported identification of thalamic nuclei by micro-electrode recordings; but in a more practical way Gaze *et al.* (1964) define the borders of the internal capsule by depth electrical recordings and audiomonitoring. The complexities of attempts to distinguish thalamic nuclei by unit and evoked potential recordings can be avoided by impedance measurements (Robinson, 1962; Robinson and Tompkins, 1964). It has been shown that the impedance of white matter is higher than that of grey, and changes of impedance are also seen from an electrode passing between brain tissue and ventricle (Fry *et al.*, 1962).

The other aids to localization can be considered as part of the process of producing a permanent lesion. The choice of the ideal physical agent for this purpose is still far from agreed. The injection of sclerosing substances has become much less popular because of the difficulty of control and the unduly large lesions often produced. Predictability of size and shape of the lesion is an obvious requirement, and from the point of view of physiological confirmation a lesion produced by reversible increments would be advantageous. An ideal lesion could be varied to correspond to the shape and inclination of the structure to be destroyed. It should not affect blood vessels passing through it and the dimensions of the electrode or probe should be small. There is also the question of expense and availability, which certainly applies to lesions made by crossfire irradiation with beams of high energy protons and by the use of ultrasonic methods. Talairach *et al.* (1960) have for many years and in a large series of cases implanted small pieces of the beta emittor ^{90}Yttrium stereotaxically. These produce constant volumes of necrosis over a period of days. The delay has the probable advantage of being less disturbing to the elderly patient than an immediate lesion but it denies all possibility of physiological control. Talairach provides this by other techniques before insertion of the isotope. In his hands the method has been strikingly successful but it has not been widely adopted.

The majority of lesions are now made by one of the following three methods: by thermo-coagulation employing a high-frequency current, by a simple cutting "leucotome", or by the use of cold with the cryogenic probe introduced during the past six years. Thermo-coagulation (Fig. 13) requires a radio-frequency generator capable of giving a constant energy output (Aronow, 1960). A uni-polar electrode has been shown to give more consistent results than a bi-polar one (Smith, 1966), and the introduction of a thermocouple

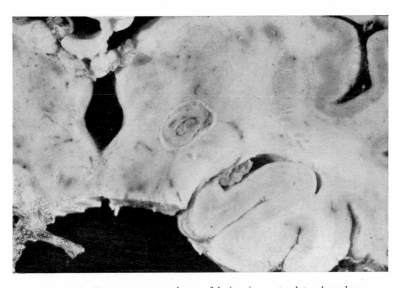

Figure 13. Post-mortem specimen of lesion in ventro-lateral nucleus produced by radio-frequency thermocoagulation (2 months after operation).

into the electrode tip permits accurate monitoring. The size and shape of the lesion depends upon the type of electrode, temperature range of application and upon certain anatomical factors. Thus, because of differences in resistance of white and grey matter and because of greater vascularization in the latter, lesions tend to expand into white matter and electrical and heat conduction and convection are influenced by the proximity of blood vessels and cerebro-spinal fluid. However, using an electrode with a stylet which can be protruded through a side-hole near its tip, it is possible to "sculpture" a lesion to a planned shape by a series of small increments in different directions (Spiegel and Wycis, 1962).

The mechanical method of producing a lesion by the use of a small "leucotome" has the virtue of simplicity and cheapness. On the introduction of such an instrument into the target area in the treatment of tremor there is often an abrupt cessation of tremor for a few seconds or half-a-minute. This "impact phenomenon" occurs on the introduction of any but the finest diameter electrode or probe and, being a type of reversible lesion, is one of the physiological aids to localization previously mentioned. Bertrand (1966) describes the use of the leucotome ". . . when tremor still persists, replacing the electrode 3 mm anteriorly or posteriorly, as the case may be, or merely opening the fine wire leukotome in either direction will interrupt tremor in one but not in the other position. Incidentally, the leukotome, although it is a rather unsophisticated instrument can be oriented to obtain temporary suppression of function medially, laterally, anteriorly or posteriorly, and thus one can determine where the lesion should actually be centered. It is essential to know in what direction centering must be corrected when this becomes necessary if one is to avoid useless and even dangerous destruction, especially if a second procedure is considered for the future." It would be natural to expect an added risk of hæmorrhage in the use of the "leucotome" but this does not appear to be the case.

The effects of cooling on nervous tissue were described by Denny-Brown et al. (1945) and by Douglas and Malcolm (1955). As an agent for reversible and permanent lesions in experimental and clinical work controllable cooling has many attractions, and techniques for this purpose were described by Dondey et al. (1961), by Mark et al. (1961) and by Cooper and Lee (1961). There was, therefore, a considerable amount of preliminary work on this subject before a suitable instrument for use in human stereotaxic surgery was introduced by the Linde Corporation in collaboration with Cooper (1965), and the basic principles of its operation are described by him as follows. "The effect of extreme cold upon biologic tissue will vary with the temperature range and rapidity of freezing rate. The temperature range employed for tissue destruction in this study has been between −50° and −100°C. The rate of freezing has been rapid, so that the freezing surface of the instrument could be cooled to −50°C within 30 seconds. The cryogenic instrument which we employ is a cannula, 2·2 mm. in diameter, which is refrigerated by liquid nitrogen. The shaft of the cannula is vacuum insulated, so that only the non-insulated tip serves as a cooling or refrigeration chamber. Liquid nitrogen, which enters the refrigeration tip under a pressure of 30 lbs and absorbs heat from the adjacent tissue, is transformed to gas and escapes through a vent supplied for this purpose. The tip temperature is monitored by an intrinsic thermocouple and the temperature is automatically controlled at a preselected level by an in-built servo-mechanism".

This technique provides many of the qualities of the ideal lesion, though there have been contradictory reports on the variability and hæmorrhagic nature of such lesions made experimentally in animal brains (Coe and Omaya, 1964; Mark *et al.*, 1965; Jinnai, 1965;

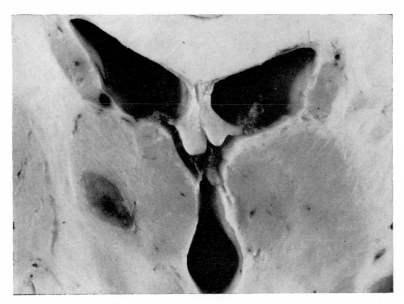

Figure 14. Post-mortem specimen of lesion in ventro-lateral nucleus produced by cryogenic instrument (5 weeks after operation).

Kandel, 1965 and Cooper, Gioino and Terry, 1965). Such dissimilar findings can only be regarded as due to differences in experimental technique. The safety of the cryogenic lesion has subsequently been demonstrated in a number of centres. Of 800 stereotaxic operations using Leksell's (1951) stereotaxic method performed by the author, the lesion (Fig. 14) has been made with the cryogenic instrument in the last 560 cases. The mortality in the first group of 240 with thermo-coagulation lesions was 2·6 per cent and in the second with cryogenic lesions was 0·9 per cent. There was a similar reduction in post-operative complications, and particularly in the occurrence of drowsiness and confusion in the post-operative period. As a result the criteria for operation were gradually extended to include patients who would previously have been excluded on the grounds of age or progression of their disease. Thus operation has been performed on eight patients over the age of 70 without mortality, the oldest being 78. Patients with serious hypertension, particularly in the presence of diabetes or with any signs of mental deterioration are still excluded. Ten patients, eight less than 60 years of age, one aged 65 and one aged 70, have had simultaneous, symmetrical, bilateral, thalamic, cryogenic lesions without any disturbance of consciousness in the post-operative period. Two were operated upon for spasmodic torticollis and eight for severe intractable pain. Similar results have been reported by Cooper who now has experience of 4,500 operations with the cryogenic instrument.

The only apparent disadvantages of the cryogenic system is the increased diameter of the probe, which is about twice that of the average electrode, and possibly the cost of the equipment. Judging both from animal and human autopsy material the lesions produced are satisfactory. In both experimental and clinical work there is a useful degree of reversibility which is seen in two situations. On impact of the probe or by preliminary cooling to $-10°C$ in the target area it is possible to assess the effect on tremor or on neighbouring structures. Perhaps even more conducive to safety, however, is the zone of disturbance of neurological function, of about 2–3 mms depth, which surrounds and precedes the expanding ice-sphere. Thus in the conscious patient adequate warning is provided of encroachment on neighbouring structures before permanent effects are produced. This is not by any means only a theoretical considera-tion and in the author's opinion is the main safety factor compared with other methods of producing stereotaxic lesions.

Anæsthesia. It is necessary to have the co-operation of the patient during the testing and production of the lesion. If general anæsthesia is used special anæsthetic agents are necessary for the first part of the operation, unless the radiological and surgical parts of the operation are performed on separate occasions, so that the patient's physical signs and co-operation are not lost subsequently. However, apart from operations on children or in the presence of violent and uncontrollable movements the author has used local anæsthesia without difficulty, the average duration of operation being about ninety minutes. Techniques requiring a longer time would probably justify the use of suitable sedation for part of the procedure. The difficulty when sedating or anæsthetizing these patients lies in making the preliminary part of the operation tolerable without removing the abnormal movements or the ability to co-operate during the final stages. In some whose movements are very violent or whose co-operation cannot be relied on even when unsedated, general anæsthesia with tracheal intubation is the simplest expedient. Other problems are posed by the stereotaxic system used. Some are more painful than others and the length of time taken varies widely. The sitting position is often associated with cardiovascular instability; recording from deep structures may be jeopardized.

Phenothiazines and pethidine in combination or singly can be used and will in large doses produce a quiet co-operative patient. There is however a risk of hypotension and of suppressing the abnormal movements. The patient may also be very inert or stuporose postoperatively. A technique using an infusion of hydroxydione (Viadril) has been described by Albe-Fessard and her colleagues (1962). This is said not to interfere with depth-recording and yet to make the operation tolerable for the patient. As described this method is an elaborate one requiring a preliminary "titration" of dose on the day preceding surgery. Useful techniques have been described by Brown (1964) who uses droperidol combined with phenoperidine, phentanyl or dextromoramide, and Coleman and de Villiers (1964) who use methobexitone (Brietal) by infusion, sometimes combined with gallamine. Methobexitone and droperidol seem to be the most useful drugs at the moment. Methobexitone given as 0·1 or 0·2 per cent infusion allows the patient to be asleep during painful procedures or at times when it is essential that he should be kept still, and to be awake or drowsy at other times. It interferes little with Parkinsonian tremor or other abnormal movements. Droperidol in doses of 5–15 mg. intramuscularly may be sufficient sedation in itself or further doses may be given intravenously. For the old and frail these methods work very well; for the young and robust and those with strong or violent movements they are not so satisfactory. The best combination seems to be methobexitone infusion after droperidol premedication. In some patients the drugs must be supplemented by physical restraint if co-operation is to be retained, and in some relatively small doses will remove abnormal movements.

APPLICATIONS

Stereotaxic surgery is used in the treatment of the following conditions:

1. Parkinson's disease.
2. Other dyskinesias.
   (a) Dystonia musculorum deformans.
   (b) Choreo-athetosis.
   (c) Idiopathic or familial tremor.
   (d) Spasmodic torticollis.
   (e) Hemiballismus.
   (f) Huntington's chorea.
   (g) Intention tremor of disseminated sclerosis.
3. Intractable or "central" pain.
4. Psychiatric conditions treatable by leucotomy.
5. Epilepsy.

PARKINSONISM

Of these conditions Parkinson's disease is by far the most frequent for which operation is undertaken, comprising about 75 per cent of the author's cases, or 603 operations on 460 patients suffering from Parkinson's disease. Parkinsonism is an extremely variable disease both as regards variety of symptomatology and rate of progression. However for the purpose of selection for operation symptoms can be considered as either "motor" or "vegetative". The motor symptoms of rigidity and tremor can be improved and frequently abolished by surgery. The vegetative symptoms of excessive salivation and perspiration, oily skin, disturbances of micturition and increased heat production are not influenced. It is fortunate that severe tremor, which almost always defies pharmacological methods, is the symptom most readily controlled surgically. Oculogyric crises are either abolished or reduced in frequency in about half the cases submitted to bilateral operation. Gillingham et al. (1964) and Cooper (1964) report similar improvement of oculogyric crises, which became apparent only after a fairly large number of bilateral operations had been performed.

Gait in Parkinson's disease is frequently disturbed in a number of different ways and has to be considered carefully in selection of patients. The common festinant gait was improved in 40 per cent and there was deterioration in 20 per cent. In these cases ataxia is the commonest cause of increasing difficulty, and if it is a significant factor initially may be a point against operation. Similarly poor gait due to true akinesia in the absence of rigidity is unlikely to be improved. In addition to propulsion and retropulsion a peculiar type of "fixation" is sometimes seen; the patient either on initiating or during walking becomes completely fixed and unable to proceed. In the presence of any of these manifestations of akinesia or brady-kinesia operation should not be recommended. Poor voice volume and severe fatiguability may also be made worse particularly after bilateral operations. But some of the apparent consequences of rigidity such as muscle pain and "weakness", and difficulty in swallowing, can be expected to improve. Relief of severe pain from rigidity is an immediate and striking benefit of reduced muscle tone. There was often an immediate reduction of postural deformities of the fingers and hand at the time the lesion was made (Gortvai 1963), accom-panied by a change to a more normal colour in the skin of the hand. It is remarkable that after many years these abnormal postures of the hand do not result in structural changes in the joints and liga-ments. Associated movements do not return although facial expres-sion may be improved. Often tremor in a hand and arm may be completely abolished yet the patient needs encouragement to remind him to use the limb, even in the absence of any detectable persisting motor or sensory defect. Handwriting looks better after the loss of tremor but it would be unwise to promise a return to employment dependent upon its quality. Improvement is seen in writing test passages, but is soon lost for anything more.

Contraindications. There are a few contraindications to stereotaxic surgery and amongst these any evidence of mental deterioration is absolute. It is necessary to be certain on this point and it may require specific enquiry from relatives or family doctor. Drug induced confusion should be recognized. Old age in itself is not a bar to operation, although, as would be expected, results of surgery are superior in the younger age groups. Amongst medical conditions, severe hypertension, diabetes and chronic pulmonary disease add considerably to the risk of operation. The former are associated with hæmorrhage at operation, and bronchopneumonia precipitated by difficulty in swallowing is the commonest cause of death in the Parkinsonian patient. As has been mentioned above, relative contra-indications appear with certain defects of voice and gait, and a patient who presents with the disease primarily exhibiting vegetative and akinetic symptoms is not a suitable subject for operation. Surgical treatment has very little to offer those with minimal tremor and whose main disability is immobility or inability to initiate movement.

The decision regarding a bedridden or institutionalized patient is usually difficult. The same general principles apply; sometimes the results are gratifying—and not always in the more promising patients. Of forty-one such patients in the author's cases, eleven became ambulant and lived more active lives in protected environments. Some of these lost a severe kyphosis and could feed themselves and perform simple tasks after varying periods of helplessness. Three cases deteriorated to the invalid state after operation and twenty-seven remained in the invalid state, although in some the pre-operative condition was appreciably improved. In selecting such patients it is important to explain the uncertainties both to relatives and patient so as to minimize possible disappointment.

Bilateral Lesions. There was some initial anxiety about the results of bilateral lesions for Parkinsonism but these have proved less hazardous than had been feared. This is in part due to improvements of technique in localization and in the use of smaller lesions. However it is prudent to be deterred by any untoward reaction on the first occasion and to make a complete reassessment of the patient's suitability before the second operation. An interval of about twelve weeks is usually allowed between the two operations, although in good risk patients with an uncomplicated first operation this is almost certainly longer than necessary. The risks and results of bilateral cases are not as favourable as in unilateral cases, mainly because the latter group contains a high proportion of the less seriously affected patients—the patient in good physical condition with unilateral Parkinson's disease presents the ideal case for surgery.

Results and Complications. Of the cases with unilateral disease tremor was abolished in 85 per cent and reduced in 10 per cent. There was recurrence of tremor in 10 per cent of cases and 6 per cent were operated on a second time for recurrence. The results as regards rigidity were generally similar, although the recurrence and re-operation rates were less.

Assessing all patients in respect of general functional ability in working or looking after themselves a system of scoring of 30 items before and after operation was used. On this basis 65 per cent were considered excellent; 25 per cent good and 10 per cent unchanged or worse.

There have been three operative deaths, two due to intracerebral hæmorrhage with death on the first and twenty-first post-operative days; and the third (a bilateral case) on insertion of the ventricular cannula at the start of the operation. A second death in 102 bilateral cases was that of a patient who became akinetic and mute after operation and died with extensive bedsores four months later.

There were five other late deaths which could be attributed to the operation.

1—Meningitis—3 months.

2—Bronchopneumonia—2 and 3 months.

2—Intracerebral hæmorrhage—10 weeks.

1—Cause unknown; died at home one month after operation.

The total mortality in 460 patients was 2 per cent (or in 603 operations = 1·5 per cent). There have been no deaths in the last 200 cases.

There are twelve patients (2·6 per cent) with permanent complications of operation as follows:

2—Hemiplegia (one with unpleasant dysthesiæ also).

3—Hemiparesis.

2—Permanent aphonia (bilateral lesions).

1—Severe hemiballismus (low thalamic lesion cured by pallidal lesion).

2—Minor forms of ballismus causing things to drop from affected hand.

2—Serious confusional states.

Transient disturbances of neurological function were recorded after 54 operations (9 per cent). These have consisted of postoperative drowsiness, confusion and speech disturbance, usually of a few days duration. There was one case of homonymous hemianopia amongst 316 lesions made through occipital burr holes. This ceased to be apparent to the patient after three weeks but a small permanent defect remains in the visual fields. Transient hemiparesis, cerebellar disturbances and ballistic movements are also included in this group.

The occurrence of ballismus-like movements following stereotaxic operations for Parkinsonism has been described by a number of writers including Dierssen et al. (1961), Gillingham et al. (1964) and Hughes (1965). This kind of abnormal movement was seen following operation in the present group of patients on twelve occasions and was of two main types, although these were probably different only in degree. Three patients showed the classical, sudden, violent shoulder muscle movements of hemiballismus. The movements started a day or two after operation and heavy sedation was necessary for their control. In two patients the movements stopped spontaneously at the end of a week and the patients made a good recovery. When the third patient's movements persisted into the second week his condition began to cause anxiety, and because of previous experience with naturally occurring hemiballismus a lesion was made in the medial globus pallidus which stopped the movements immediately. The other type consisted of a much milder disorder which was annoying to the patient because the occasional unexpected jerk of the arm caused the hand to drop or throw anything held in it. Of nine patients, five recovered in periods up to three months but four patients are still troubled by this complication. There seems no doubt that in these cases the extent of the lesion has been excessive in a ventral direction towards or involving the subthalamic nucleus, although with the disappearance of ballistic movements all these patients have had excellent results as regards tremor and rigidity. Using a subthalamic target in the treatment of Parkinsonism Andy et al. (1963) produced hemiballismus of this type in five of fifty-eight patients.

The most persistent and troublesome widely reported complication of bilateral thalamic lesions for Parkinsonism is speech disturbance. This consists of reduction in voice volume sometimes amounting to aphonia and gross dysarthria with occasionally an apparent word-blocking, though without true dysphasia. When speech is normal before the second operation 25 per cent of patients show some disturbance subsequently but this is in most cases recoverable in the course of a few weeks. Patients with an existing serious defect of speech run a 50 per cent risk of this being made worse by a bilateral operation and in the light of these findings operation as at present performed should usually be withheld in such cases. The general incidence of complications is nearly doubled following a lesion on the second side. This is partly arithmetical as regards number of operations and total size of lesion and partly due to the poorer condition of patients with bilateral disease. In two patients troublesome dysphagia was seen after a second operation and Gillingham (1966) mentions impotence under similar circumstances. It is not at all uncommon to see some slight recurrence of tremor on the first side at the time of making the lesion on the second side. This is a similar phenomenon to the initiation or aggravation of tremor on one side previously minimally affected or unaffected as a lesion relieves the opposite limbs, and can be seen to occur on the operating table.

Post-operative rehabilitation is an essential part of treatment, particularly since patients not infrequently show a reluctance to make use of limbs which have been freed from rigidity and tremor. This sometimes amounts to an apparent "unawareness" of the limb. On the day after operation physiotherapy should begin including walking exercises, and as pointed out by Hurwitz (1964) patients should be encouraged to become mobile again no matter how crippled they were by the disease prior to operation. It is important to supervise a patient's progress after his return home because over-anxious relatives sometimes press him into a state of continued invalidism at a time when he should be encouraged to increasing activity. In most cases anti-Parkinson medication should be continued and sudden cessation of drug therapy is inadvisable. Sometimes dosage can be reduced and this in itself may contribute to the patient's well-being.

Site and Size of Lesions. Lesions in the treatment of Parkinson's disease were first made in the ansa lenticularis and in the medial

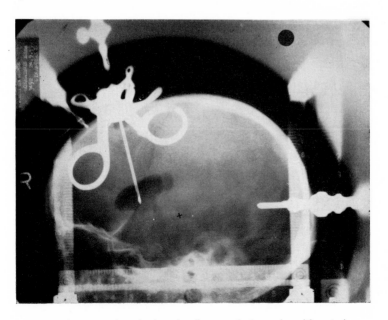

Figure 15. Lateral projection showing ventriculography with anterior and posterior commissures pinpointed and cross marking position of target. (Leksell's instrument.)

globus pallidus (Spiegel and Wycis, 1950) but most surgeons now use a target in or including part of the ventro-lateral nucleus of the thalamus contralateral to the affected limbs. This area was first suggested by Hassler (1955). Thalamic operations were then performed by Riechert in association with Hassler on the theoretical basis of reduction of corticofugal impulses to the skeletal muscles by destruction of thalamo-cortical projections from the ventrolateral nucleus, as discussed by Hassler *et al.* in their paper (1960). Cooper and Bravo (1958) also suggested a similar thalamic target as a result of an analysis of site of lesion and results obtained in their previous large series of operations. Lesions have been made in both the anterior and posterior parts of the nucleus (ventralis oralis anterior and posterior: VOA and VOP of Hassler). A spherical lesion situated ventrally in VOP and reached from a postero-frontal burr hole has been used in the last 300 of the cases described in this account. A similar number was treated previously with a cylindrical lesion involving both VOA and VOP at a more dorsal level by an electrode introduced through an occipital burr hole. The present lesion is

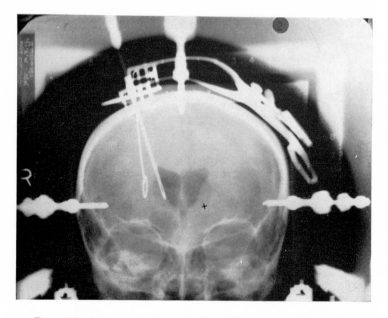

Figure 16. Antero-posterior projection with cross showing position of target.

centered by radiological localization at the junction of the posterior and middle thirds of the line joining the anterior and posterior commissures as seen on the lateral view of the third ventricle (Fig. 15). In the antero-posterior projection the centre of the target area is on average thirteen millimetres from a midline passing through the septum lucidum and the third ventricle (Fig. 16). The lesion produced is a sphere 6 mms in diameter, causing destruction of approximately 100 c.mm of tissue. In dealing with violent tremors of wide excursion a larger lesion is required, and this is achieved by a further over-lapping lesion anterior to the first, converting the sphere into an ovoid. The posterior positioning of the first lesion can be judged by the patient's complaint of dysthesiæ, usually in the thumb, index and middle finger and at the angle of the mouth as a cryogenic lesion is completed. This immediately disappears on reheating. Too medial a lesion will fail to influence tremor in the leg and foot and this can be corrected by replacing the probe 2 mms laterally.

It need hardly be pointed out that the object of surgery is to produce the minimum destruction compatible with a permanent relief of symptoms, particularly in operations on the frail and aged and when bilateral lesions are indicated. This ideal is for most surgeons the result of experience, as there is a strong inclination to decrease lesion size until an increasing recurrence rate becomes apparent. As a result of such experiences and as suggested by Gillingham et al. (1964) and by Walsh (1966), lesions of 100–150 c.mm appear to be a satisfactory compromise.

Surgeons have usually tried to avoid damage to the internal capsule, fearing serious motor or sensory deficits. Guiot et al. (1960), Jinnai et al. (1961), and Gillingham (1962) deliberately include the adjacent capsule in both thalamic and pallidal lesions. By detailed physiological studies of the internal capsule during stereotaxic operations Gillingham has also developed a technique for producing small lesions in the posterior limb of the capsule itself, quite separately from thalamic lesions. There seems no doubt of the localization nor of the therapeutic value of such lesions and further information concerning the detailed constitution of the capsule can be expected from this work.

Spiegel et al. (1962) described the production of lesions as re-stricted as far as possible to Forel's field H at the cephalad and lateral aspects of the red nucleus. This procedure they have called "campo-tomy" and by it they can interrupt a large proportion of pallido-fugal fibres to the red nucleus and reticular formation and can also divide cerebello-thalamopallidal fibres with less risk to cortico-fugal fibres than with the usual lesions adjacent to the capsule. They place the lesion medial to the corpus Luysii to avoid damage to this structure and in some cases add lesions in the thalamus above Forel's field. Spiegel *et al.* (1963) showed good results of lesions of field H and stated that the effect on tremor and rigidity was more pronounced following lesions of the thalamic part of field H in front of and lateral to the red nucleus than following lesions in the mesencephalic part. The complication rate appeared similar to that associated with posterior VL lesions. Andy *et al.* (1963) studied 58 patients undergoing 72 diencephalic operations for tremor and concluded: "that the optimum area for the most efficient lesion was in the posterior subthalamus and included the field H of Forel, zona incerta and the prerubral field medial to the subthalamic nuclei. Both the short and long-lasting complications following lesions placed in the optimum site of the subthalamus were not as pronounced as those associated with lesions in other areas studied." Strassburger and French (1961) reported a series of experiments in 1960 and 1961 on Serpasil-induced tremor in cats. Stereotaxic lesions were then placed in a number of structures. Lesions in three areas were effective in modifying induced tremor in the contralateral limbs; namely, globus pallidus, thalamic ventro-lateral nucleus and Forel's field H. Of these, under experimental conditions in the cat, lesions of Forel's field appeared to be the most effective. The results of subthalamic lesions in a series of fifty patients are given in a recent communication by Story *et al.* (1965).

Some workers have had an undesirable frequency of complications with subthalamic lesions and this led Adams and Rutkin (1965), following the suggestion of Schulman (1957) and the work of Rand *et al.* (1962), to make lesions in the *centre médian*. This nucleus has also been included in lesions for the dyskinesias by Cooper (1965) and for intractable pain by Talairach *et al.* (1949), as will be described later. The theoretical basis of this work depends on the existence of projections on to the nucleus from the globus pallidus and from the precentral motor cortex. Specific afferent fibres to the putamen arise in the *centre médian* and some somatosensory fibres pass through it. It is interesting that in this site also the authors produced results in a small series (26 patients) which are comparable with those obtained from lesions in the other situations which have been described.

The motivation of this widespread search for lesion sites in the treatment of Parkinsonism and the other dyskinesias is partly positive and in part negative in the avoidance of undesirable side effects. The extent over which effective lesions have been reported was described as follows by Kjellberg (1965): "the lesions extend nearly the full distance from the anterior to the posterior commissures. In general, lesions extend below the inter-commissural line about 5 mm in the anterior third and to about 10 mm above the line through its length. In the antero-posterior view, lesions lie between 10 and 20 mm lateral to the midline or from the plane going through the lateral edge of the lateral ventricle to about half way closer to the midline. This is a remarkably broad zone. An average of inter-commissural lengths given by Spiegel and Wycis is 24·8 mm, by Talairach is 25 mm; the total volume of this effective zone is then about 3 cubic centimetres. Included in it are the medial half of the globus pallidus, the anterior half of the internal capsule with the interlacing fibres of the fasciculus lenticularis, and the extralaminar thalamic nuclei; in Walker's terminology ventralis anterior (VA), ventralis lateralis (VL), ventralis posterior (VP), and the centrum medianum (CM)."

Kjellberg deals attractively with the twin problems of a super-imposed lesion restoring apparent neurological normality and the large volume of brain in which this can be achieved by compara-tively small lesions—problems which will continue to stimulate widespread physiological, clinical and dialectical activity.

OTHER DYSKINESIAS

A further problem, in addition to the two mentioned in the last paragraph, is posed by the non-specific nature of these lesions in relation to the site and nature of the pathological process. Thus, by lesions similar in situation to those described in the section on Parkinson's disease, a considerable number of successes have been recorded in the treatment of the varied states of hyperkinesia listed earlier in this chapter. The most comprehensive account of the recent surgical treatment of these conditions is given by Cooper (1965). This describes experience of 110 cases of intention tremor (familial, "benign", disseminated sclerosis etc.); 130 cases of dystonia muscu-lorum deformans and 75 cases of spasmodic torticollis or retrocollis, which are regarded by Cooper as variants of dystonia.

Intention Tremor. Cooper reports abolition of this symptom in 90 per cent of cases by a contralateral lesion involving the anterior portion of the ventro-postero-lateral and ventro-postero-medial nuclei and the posterior portion of the ventro-lateral nucleus. In the dyskinesias Cooper employs a larger lesion than in Parkinson's disease involving sensory nuclei and including *centre médian* in dystonic conditions. Other workers prefer lesions in the subthalamic region, as described above. There is little difficulty in case selection except in disseminated sclerosis. The widespread destruction in this disease is demonstrable at ventriculography by extreme ventricular dilatation, and the possibility of untoward side effects is correspondingly increased. There is in any case little to be gained by operation unless intention tremor is a major cause of the patient's disability, implying the retention of sufficient useful motor function in the absence of tremor. The number of cases of disseminated sclerosis for which surgery is indicated is small.

Dystonia Musculorum Deformans includes probably the most important group of patients as this usually progressive and extremely disabling disease can be favourably influenced in a high proportion of cases. Dystonia is a disorder superimposed in childhood or in early adult life on a previously normal motor system, in contrast to choreo-athetosis which is usually associated with spasticity and paralysis from birth or infancy. Abnormal movements may be eliminated in the latter group but, as was suggested in the treatment of disseminated sclerosis, there is little gained if the patient remains incapable of useful activity. This is particularly so in children of low I.Q. However, Narabayashi *et al.*, 1960; Narabayashi, 1962, have reported a series of 169 patients suffering from "infantile cerebral palsy" subjected to pallidal and subsequently to thalamic operations. They were all of the type in which improvement rather than cure could be hoped for, and 78 per cent were said to have shown some amelioration of such symptoms as facial grimacing, protrusion of the tongue, extensor spasms of the shoulder muscles, abdominal respiration, scissor legs and inverted legs. Cooper reports success in 70 per cent of dystonic cases using bilateral comma-shaped lesions destroying the posterior half of the ventro-lateral nucleus, the anterior portions of ventralis posterolateralis and medialis and the outer two-thirds of *centre médian*. Many of these young patients have had very large bilateral thalamic lesions and have shown no signs of intellectual or emotional damage over long periods of observation. Such resilience is limited to the youthful brain and is most definitely lost in the adult.

The theoretical basis for including sensory nuclei is the apparent initiation of dystonic responses secondary to voluntary movements of the extremities which is aggravated or facilitated by diverse proprioceptive or loading stimuli. Although there is a maximal contra-lateral effect, bilateral lesions are usually necessary in treating dystonic conditions even when the clinical manifestations are predominantly unilateral. Occasionally a good result follows a unilateral lesion which improves the condition bilaterally, although the ipsilateral improvement may not be maintained. Usually in the treatment of Parkinsonian tremor and rigidity and tremor of other ætiologies the maximum effect is seen at the time of the infliction of the lesion. Sometimes with bilateral lesions for Parkinson's disease improvement continues over a period of months (Gillingham *et al.*, 1964). This is also true with dystonia, when gradual improvement may continue for a considerable period of time with physiotherapy. Conversely after an initial decrease in abnormal movements a recurrence or progression of the condition may be seen. It is the author's impression, from personal experience and from the literature in English, that Cooper's results in the treatment of dyskinesias are superior to those obtained by most surgeons. This can in part be attributed to his very extensive experience, leading to the production of larger bilateral lesions in the sensorimotor elements of the thalamus in a predominantly youthful group. There seems no doubt that large thalamic lesions are required, although Spiegel *et al.* (1963) and Mundinger (1965) have reported successes with small sub-thalamic lesions ("campotomy").

Spasmodic Torticollis or Retrocollis. Although many cases appear to be localized forms of dystonia the results of stereotaxic operations for this condition have usually been disappointing and the success rate lower than in dystonic cases. A frequent experience has been recurrence after initial improvement. Cooper (1965) in the publication previously referred to in this section, shows some gratifying results of extensive bilateral thalamic lesions, as used by him in dystonia. The lesions are monitored by EMG recordings from the affected nuchal musculature and there are striking examples of cessation of unilateral involuntary muscular activity only on completion of bilateral lesions. The author's experience of the treatment of nine cases of this condition has been discouraging.

Hemiballismus has been considered as a comparatively rare complication of thalamic surgery. Occasionally the naturally occurring condition is sufficiently severe to warrant an attempt to control it by stereotaxic surgery. Such patients are usually in poor condition for surgery being often arteriopathic and hypertensive, apart from the distress and exhaustion caused by the ballistic movements. It is, fortunately, usually possible to stop the movements completely by a contralateral pallidal or thalamic lesion.

Huntington's Chorea was the condition for which stereotaxic surgery was first performed by Spiegel and Wycis (1950) in 1948. The abnormal movements in this condition are not difficult to reduce or abolish by either pallidal or thalamic lesions and bilateral lesions are well tolerated. The operation is performed to enable the patient to feed himself or to hold a paper and perform simple tasks and to reduce the difficulties of nursing. It is hardly justified to submit the advanced demented case to such procedures.

PAIN

Attempts to control intractable pain by stereotaxic surgery have been directed to three sites—the mesencephalon, the thalamus, and the parietal lobe. The type of pain demanding such operations is either severe pain of malignant origin such as carcinoma involving the maxilla or base of the skull, which for anatomical reasons cannot be dealt with by other neurosurgical procedures; or pain of a "central" type originating or being perpetuated in the central nervous system such as the thalamic syndrome of Dejerine and Roussy (1906), painful phantoms, post-herpetic neuralgia and "atypical" facial pain (pain of unknown ætiology not fulfilling the diagnostic criteria of classical trigeminal neuralgia).

The results of mesencephalic tractotomy by stereotaxic means have been described by Spiegel and Wycis (1953), Mazars et al. (1960), and recently by Helfant, Leksell and Strang (1965). The lesions interrupt spino- and trigemino-thalamic tracts. Relief of pain was obtained in about half the patients, mostly in the later stages of malignancy with short post-operative survival periods. There was a high proportion of neurological complications of which the most distressing was the development of uncomfortable dysæsthesiæ—a constant risk in any type of mesencephalic tractotomy.

Cortical resections of portions of the parietal lobe have been performed in the treatment of painful phantoms and other painful conditions by Gutierrez-Mahoney (1944), Lhermitte and Puech (1946) and others. In a very full study of cortical and subcortical stimulation in a case of a painful phantom arm Pertuiset et al. (1959) concluded that electrical stimulation of the postcentral gyrus evokes pain only when the extremity is spontaneously painful. White and Sweet (1955) reviewed this type of surgery and expressed the view that cortical sensory representation of the limbs is too diffuse to permit resections of sufficient extent to give lasting relief of phantom pain. Talairach et al. (1960) have, however, employed a rather elaborate stereotaxic technique of stimulation, recording and production of localized lesions outside the foot of the corona radiata. In these cases of painful phantom the painful sensations were reproduced by stimulation under local anæsthesia and on some occasions patients reported simultaneous temporary changes in the size, shape and position of the phantom. Accurate radiological localization of the major cortical fissures outlining the parietal lobe has been developed in this work and Talairach's technique enables him to stimulate and record from a number of fine electrodes passed into the parietal lobe. This region of the corona radiata, lying above the Sylvian fissure and deep to the secondary sensory area of Penfield, not only comprises fibres running from thalamus to post-central sensory cortex and the second sensory area but also the diffuse association pathways to the frontal lobe and elsewhere in the brain. Talairach suggests that it seems sufficient to introduce a functional disturbance into this complex system to modify the patients' experience of pain. Pathways with an antero-posterior somatotopic organization of the face to the leg similar to that of the primary sensory cortex have been demonstrated by these workers. In the cases described lesions were made either by thermo-coagulation or by implantation of ^{90}Yttrium at the site where stimulation elicited sensory phenomena in the painful area. Seven out of eight patients lost their pain. In one patient pain persisted in an area which had not been activated on stimulation. On a second occasion the appropriate site of stimulation was found and the pain relieved. The patients did not show sensory defects of astereognosis and spatial disorientation after operation as would be expected after resections of parietal cortex. These experiences lend some support to the views of Biemond (1956) on cortical pain mechanisms.

Thalamic lesions for painful conditions were described soon after the introduction of stereotaxic surgery. Talairach et al. (1949) reported twelve cases of the thalamic syndrome treated with lesions in ventralis posterolateralis or medialis on the side opposite to the pain. Hécaen et al. (1949) described improved results in cases in which a lesion in centre médian was added. This first emphasized the distinction between the specific somæsthetic pathways and the diffuse spino-reticular-thalamic system. At the thalamic level these are represented respectively by a lateral group of nuclei (VPL and VPM) and by a medial group (centre médian and the intralaminar nuclei). Bowsher (1957) points out "the very small number of pain fibres reaching the specific thalamic nucleus in comparison with the very large number of fibres from the medial leminiscus." Glees and Bailey (1951) state that the direct spino-thalamic tract contains only 1,500 medullated fibres at the level of the superior colliculus.

All reports on the results of thalamic surgery for pain have shown a considerable rate of recurrence after a high proportion of relief initially. Attempts to explain this have included a gradual recovery of function of neurological elements in the vicinity of the lesion and the presence of bilateral pathways. In order to increase the size of the lesion safely and to deal with the first possibility, Mark and his co-workers (Mark *et al.*, 1960, 1962; Ervin and Mark 1964) implanted thalamic electrodes which were left in position for periods of months, so that further coagulations could be made as seemed necessary. Although the therapeutic results are difficult to evaluate, physiological studies associated with these procedures are of considerable interest. Evoked potential studies showed short latency responses with a somatotopic distribution in the lateral group of nuclei. However, in the medial nuclei following the short latency response prolonged rhythmic activity was seen projecting to the cortex. Pethidine enhanced the evoked response in the lateral nuclei while it diminished that of the medial nuclei and abolished the rhythmic after-discharge. It was suggested that the non-specific medial group of nuclei may be responsible for the experience of pain. Certainly relief of pain can be achieved by thalamic lesions without demonstrable analgesia or other sensory loss, and stimulation in the lateral specific nuclei does not produce painful responses. It seems possible that some painful syndromes may be relieved by lesions confined to the diffuse system, by medially placed thalamic lesions sparing the specific nuclei and avoiding additional neurological deficits.

A further approach to the prevention of recurrence of pain has been by the production of bilateral lesions. It was feared on theoretical grounds that bilateral lesions of the diffuse, non-specific system could so reduce reticular sensory input as to interfere with consciousness. This fear has proved to be unjustified. Bilateral lesions consisting of 6 mm spheres inflicted with the cryogenic instrument have been produced on ten occasions with no disturbance of consciousness. Previously (Hankinson, 1961) eighteen patients had had unilateral thalamic lesions for pain. The twenty-eight patients were classified as follows:

"Thalamic syndrome"	9
Post-herpetic neuralgia	4
Intercostal neuralgia	1
Spinal cord pain (myelitis, tabes etc.)	5
Carcinoma involving skull (antrum, post-nasal space etc.)	5
Atypical facial pain	3
Carcinoma of uterus—sciatic pain	1

The second group of patients with simultaneous bilateral lesions involving nucleus parafascicularis lying between the wall of the third ventricle and nucleus *centre médian* and CM itself have shown a considerable improvement and at present the operation appears to be justified in some patients in which all else has failed. It is not always possible to exclude "psychogenic" pains and, as might be expected, they successfully defy all efforts for their relief. With the lesions described the painful malignant conditions of the head and neck have all been relieved, although the longest survival was fifteen months and the shortest three months. Three cases of ophthalmic post-herpetic neuralgia were considerably relieved, but two were left with a small painful area, about 1 cm in diameter at the lateral corner of the orbit. Four of the cases of "thalamic syndrome" have had considerable reduction in attacks of spontaneous pain, two having been free of attacks for one year and eighteen months respectively.

It might seem that the beneficial results of these operations, devoid as they usually are of any persistent sensory deficit, could be attributed to a "leucotomy" effect. It is true that euphoria is described in the post-operative period in five patients but in the six submitted to psychiatric examination no changes comparable with those of leucotomy were apparent. Bilateral lesions involving the dorso-median nuclei will produce the most profound psychiatric disturbance, comparable with the effects of a radical, classical pre-frontal leucotomy. Such patients, as is well known, lose their emotional response to pain, which they affirm they still feel. The patients just described, operated upon for pains of the face and skull, subsequently denied having pain and showed no sensory loss but were otherwise unchanged. This may represent, in successful cases, an adequate, if rather fortuitous disturbance of the slow-conducting pain pathways of the diffuse spino-reticular-thalamic system, but further information is required before any firm conclusions can be drawn in this rather speculative field.

PSYCHOSURGERY

Reference has already been made to the effects on personality of lesions involving the dorso-median nuclei of the thalamus as reported by Spiegel and Wycis (1952). Leksell's stereotaxic method (1949) was employed in 116 cases described by Herner (1961). Bilateral frontal lesions interrupting the fronto-thalamic radiations were made in 64 patients suffering from schizophrenia, 19 depressive states, 15 anxiety neurosis and 18 obsessional neurosis. Good results were obtained in 34 per cent of patients, fair in 45 per cent and poor in 21 per cent. Within two years of operation 40 per cent of 79 institutionalized patients were discharged home. Epilepsy occurred in 4 patients (3·4 per cent).

Knight (1965) recently introduced a stereotaxic technique for a modified type of orbital undercutting. Using McCaul's stereotaxic device (1959) to introduce seeds of ^{90}Yttrium a lesion was planned confined to the posterior 2 cm of the original undercutting incision in the substantia innominata, underlying cortical area 13, and situated 1 cm from the midline at its medial edge and 1 cm above the orbital roof. The posterior margin lies only 0·5 cm anterior to the plane of the tuberculum sellæ. Two rows of four seeds each were laid on each side resulting in a flat lesion no more than 5 mms in thickness. Good results were also obtained in some cases later in the series when the outer row of seeds near the fronto-thalamic tract was omitted. No deaths occurred in 90 stereotaxic operations; there was a mortality of 1·3 per cent in 554 surgical undercutting operations. There was a 10 per cent incidence of epilepsy by the surgical method and 3 per cent by stereotaxis. Depression was strikingly improved by the stereotaxic operation and good results were obtained in obsessional and anxiety states. It is preferable to the surgical procedure in patients of advanced years and poor physical condition.

EPILEPSY

Riechert and Hassler (1957), Baird, Spiegel and Wycis (1960), Talairach et al (1962) and Bancaud et al (1965), have all reported stereotaxic operations for epilepsy. The technique involves multiple depth recordings and destruction of apparent foci of origin of epileptic discharge. Talairach's work is basically the same as that described in connection with his operations for pain. Recent papers have been concerned with the treatment of temporal lobe epilepsy. Turner (1963) described 38 cases of psychomotor or mixed epilepsy treated by unilateral or bilateral section of the temporal lobe isthmus in the roof of the temporal horn. These lesions were made freehand with the leucotome but in subsequent cases (1966) radio-frequency coagulation and Hughes' stereotaxic instrument (1961) have been employed. Depth electrode recordings were found less helpful than sphenoidal electrodes using pentothal anæsthesia. The value of this procedure lies in the blocking of bilaterally occurring discharges by lesions in white matter without cortical destruction—the difference between "lobotomy" and "lobectomy". It was found that lobotomy of the temporal lobe isthmus greatly improved major psychomotor attacks and the temperamental disturbances of uncontrollable rage or fear, and improved grand mal to some extent. No deficit of intellect or memory was found after any of these procedures.

Narabayashi *et al.* (1963) present the results of stereotaxic oil-wax destruction of the amygdaloid nucleus in 39 patients unilaterally and in 21 patients bilaterally. All had severe behaviour disorders and 46 suffered from clinical epilepsy. Eight of the 14 non-epileptics had EEG abnormalities. The striking finding in this series of patients was the high (85 per cent) improvement in behaviour and the low (10 per cent) response as regards epilepsy. Again there were no disturbances of memory or signs and symptoms suggesting the Klüver-Bucy syndrome (disturbance of memory, emotion and sexual behaviour), even after bilateral amygdaloid destruction.

Talairach and Szikla (1965) performed partial amygdalo-hippo-campal destruction by ^{90}Yttrium in 14 cases of intractable temporal lobe epilepsy. Ten patients had minimal disturbances of memory and concentration which disappeared in two months. More serious memory disorders were seen in two patients with bilateral lesions. Epileptic attacks ceased in nine patients. Of nine with behaviour disorders, six were improved and three unchanged. As might be expected from their previous experience these authors are strongly in favour of depth-electrode studies as a guide to the production of lesions and in order to limit operation to primary temporal lobe abnormalities.

The therapeutic range of stereotaxic surgery is wide although the prospects of success that can be expected vary considerably from one condition to another. In the investigation of normal and abnormal human neural mechanisms the opportunities furnished by stereotaxic operations in the conscious patient are unrivalled. The quality of personnel and equipment required for this work is no less than that demanded in the neuro-physiological laboratory and, where this is adequate, the method can be expected to produce important fundamental information.

References

ADAMS, J. E., and RUTKIN, B. B. (1965). *Confin. neurol.*, **26**, 231.

ALBE-FESSARD, D., ARFEL, G., GUIOT, G., HARDY, J., VOURC'H, G., HERTZOG, E., ALEONARD, P., and DEROME, P. (1962). *Rev. neurol.*, **106**, 89.

ANDY, O. J., JURKO, M. F., and SIAS, F. R. (1963). *J. Neurosurg.*, **20**, 860.

ARONOW, S. (1960). *J. Neurosurg.*, **17**, 431.

BAIRD, H. W. III., SPIEGEL, E. A., and WYCIS, H. T. (1960). *Confin. neurol.*, **20**, 26.

BANCAUD, J., TALAIRACH, J., BONIS, A., SCHAUB, C., SZIKLA, G., MOREL, P., and BORDAS-FERRER, M. (1965). *La stéréoélectroencéphalographie dans l'épilepsie.*, Paris; Masson.

BERTRAND, C. (1966). 2nd Symp. Parkinson's Dis. Supplement *J. Neurosurg.*, **24,** 446.

BIEMOND, A. (1956). *Arch. Neurol. Psychiat.*, **75,** 231.

BOWSHER, D. (1957). *Brain*, **80,** 606.

BROWN, A. S. (1964). *Anæsthesia*, **19,** 70.

COE, J., and OMAYA, A. K. (1964). *J. Neurosurg.*, **21,** 433.

COLEMAN, D. J., and VILLIERS, V. C. DE. (1964). *Anæsthesia*, **19,** 60.

COOPER, I. S. (1964). *J. Amer. Geriat. Soc.*, **12,** 813.

COOPER, I. S. (1965). *J. Neurol. Sci.*, **2,** 493.

COOPER, I. S., and BRAVO, G. J. (1958). *Neurology.*, **8,** 701.

COOPER, I. S., GIOINO, G., and TERRY, R. (1965). *Confin neurol.*, **26,** 161.

COOPER, I. S., and LEE, A. J. (1961). *J. Nerv. and Ment. Dis.*, **133,** 259.

DEJERINE, J., and ROUSSY, G. (1906). *Rev. neurol.*, **14,** 521.

DELMAS, A., and PERTUISET, B. (1959). *La topométrie cranio-encéphalique chez l'homme.* Springfield, Ill.: Charles C. Thomas; Paris; Masson.

DENNY-BROWN, D., ADAMS, R. D., BRENNE, C., and DOHERTY, M. M. (1945). *J. Neuropath. exp. Neurol.*, **4,** 305.

DIERSSEN, G., GIOINO, G., and COOPER, I. S. (1961). *Neurology*, **11,** 894.

DONDEY, M., ALBE-FESSARD, D., and LE BEAU, J. (1961). *Rev. neurol.*, **105,** 186.

DOUGLAS, W. W., and MALCOLM, J. L. (1955). *J. Physiol.*, **130,** 63.

ERVIN, F. R., and MARK, V. H. (1964). *Ann. N.Y. Acad. Sci.*, **112,** 81.

FRY, W. J., FRY, F. J., LEICHNER, G. H., and HEIMBURGER, R. F. (1962). *J. Neurosurg.*, **19,** 793.

GAZE, R. M., GILLINGHAM, F. J., KALYANARAMAN, S., PORTER, R. W., DONALD-SON, A. A., and DONALDSON, I. M. L. (1964). *Brain*, **87,** 691.

GILLINGHAM, F. J. (1962). *Confin. neurol.*, **22,** 385.

GILLINGHAM, F. J. (1966). 2nd Symp. Parkinson's Dis. Supplement *J. Neurosurg.*, **24,** 473.

GILLINGHAM, F. J., KALYANARAMAN, S., and DONALDSON, A. A. (1964). *Brit. med. J.*, **2,** 656.

GLEES, P., and BAILEY, R. A. (1951). *Mschr. Psychiat. Neurol.*, **122,** 129.

GORTVAI, P. (1963). *J. Neurol. Neurosurg. Psychiat.*, **26,** 33.

GUIOT, G., BRION, S., FARDEAU, M., BETTAIEB, A., and MOLINA, P. (1960). *Rev. neurol.*, **102,** 220.

GUTIERREZ-MAHONY, C. G. (1944). *J. Neurosurg.*, **1,** 156.

HANKINSON, J. (1960). *Postgrad. med. J.*, **36,** 242.

HANKINSON, J. (1961). *Proc. roy. Soc. Med.*, **54,** 380.

HASSLER, R. (1955). *Proc. 2nd Int. Congr. Neuropath. (London).* Amsterdam, *Excerpta Medica. Pt. I*, 29.

HASSLER, R., RIECHERT, T., MUNDINGER, F., UMBACH, W., and GANGLBERGER, J. A. (1960). *Brain*, **83,** 337.

HÉCAEN, H., TALAIRACH, J., DAVID, M., and DELL, M. B. (1949). *Rev. neurol.*, **81,** 817.

HELFANT, M. H., LEKSELL, L., and STRANG, R. R. (1965). *Acta chir. scand.*, **129,** 573.

HERNER, T. (1961). *Acta psychiat. scand.*, **36,** Supp. 158.

HORSLEY, V., and CLARKE, R. H. (1908). *Brain*, **31,** 45.

HUGHES, B. (1961). "Stereotactic Surgery," in *British Surgical Practice: Surgical Progress.* London, Butterworths.

HUGHES, B. (1965). *J. Neurol. Neurosurg. Psychiat.*, **28,** 291.

HURWITZ, L. J. (1964). *Lancet*, **2,** 953.

JASPER, H., and BERTRAND, G. (1965). *Arch. Neurol. (Chicago)*, **12**, 445.

JINNAI, D. (1965). *Confin. neurol.*, **26**, 437.

JINNAI, D., NISHIMOTO, A., MATSUMOTO, K., and HANDA, S. (1961). (2nd Int. Congr. Neurol. Surg., Washington D.C.). *Excerpta Med.*, **36**, E94.

KANDEL, E. I. (1965). *Confin. neurol.*, **26**, 306.

KJELLBERG, R. N. (1965). *Confin. neurol.*, **26**, 328.

KNIGHT, G. C. (1965). *J. Neurol. Neurosurg. Psychiat.*, **28**, 304.

LEKSELL, L. (1951). *Acta chir. scand.*, **102**, 316.

LHERMITTE, J., and PUECH, P. (1946). *Rev. neurol.*, **78**, 33.

MCCAUL, I. R. (1959). *J. Neurol. Neurosurg. Psychiat.*, **22**, 109.

MARK, V. H., CHATO, J. C., EASTMAN, F. G., ARONOW, S., and ERVIN, F. R. (1961). *Science*, **134**, 1520.

MARK, V. H., CHIBA, T., ERVIN, F. R., and HAMLIN, H. (1965). *Confin. neurol.*, **26**, 178.

MARK, V. H., ERVIN, F. R., and HACKETT, T. P. (1960). *Arch. neurol.*, **3**, 351.

MARK, V. H., ERVIN, F. R., and YAKOVLEV, P. J. (1962). *Confin. neurol.*, **22**, 238.

MAZARS, G., ROGE, R., and PANSINI, A. (1960). *J. Neurol. Neurosurg. Psychiat.*, **23**, 352.

MUNDINGER, F. (1965). *Confin. neurol.*, **26**, 222.

NARABAYASHI, H. (1962). *Confin. neurol.*, **22**, 364.

NARABAYASHI, H., NAGAO, T., SAITO, Y., YOSHIDA, M., and NAGAHATA, M. (1963). *Arch. Neurol.*, **9**, 1.

NARABAYASHI, H., SHIMAZU, H., FUJITA, Y., SHIKIBA, S., NAGAO, T., and NAGAHATA, M. (1960). *Neurology. (Minneap.)*, **10**, 61.

PERTUISET, J., HIRSCH, F., CALVERT, J., and LEFRANC, E. (1959). *Rev. neurol.*, **101**, 140.

RAND, R. W., CRANDALL, P. H., ADEY, W. R., WALTER, R. D., and MARKHAM, C. H. (1962). *Neurology (Minneap.)*, **12**, 754.

RIECHERT, T., and HASSLER, R. (1957). *Acta neurochir.*, **5**, 330.

ROBINSON, B. W. (1962). *Exp. Neurol.*, **6**, 201.

ROBINSON, B. W., and TOMPKINS, H. E. (1964). *Arch. Neurol. (Chic.)*, **10**, 563.

SCHALTENBRAND, G., and BAILEY, P. (Ed.). (1959). *Introduction to Stereotaxis with an Atlas of the Human Brain*. 3 vols. Stuttgart, Thieme.

SCHULMAN, S. (1957). *J. Neuropath. exp. Neurol.*, **16**, 446.

SMITH, M. C. (1966). 2nd Symp. Parkinson's Dis. Supplement *J. Neurosurg.*, **24**, 443.

SPIEGEL, E. A. (1965). *Confin. neurol.*, **26**, 125.

SPIEGEL, E. A., and WYCIS, H. T. (1950). *Arch. Neurol. Psychiat. (Chic.)*, **64**, 295.

SPIEGEL, E. A., and WYCIS, H. T. (1952). "Stereoencephalotomy (thalamotomy and related procedures)." Part I. *Methods and Stereotaxis Atlas of the Human Brain*, New York, Grune & Stratton.

SPIEGEL, E. A., and WYCIS, H. T. (1962). "Stereoencephalotomy (thalamotomy and related procedures)." Part II. *Clinical and Physiological Applications.* New York, Grune & Stratton.

SPIEGEL, E. A., and WYCIS, H. T. (1953). *Arch. Neurol. Psychiat. (Chic.)*, **69**, 1.

SPIEGEL, E. A., WYCIS, H. T., MARKS, M., and LEE, A. J. (1947). *Science*, **106**, 349.

SPIEGEL, E. A., WYCIS, H. T., SZEKELY, E. G., BAIRD, H. W. III., ADAMS, J., and FLANAGAN, M. (1962). *Trans. Amer. neurol. Ass.*, **87**, 240.

SPIEGEL, E. A., WYCIS, H. T., SZEKELY, E. G., ADAMS, J., FLANAGAN, M., and BAIRD, H. W. III. (1963). *J. Neurosurg.*, **20**, 771.

STORY, J. L., FRENCH, L. A., CHOU, S. N., and MEIER, M. J. (1965). *Confin. neurol.*, **26**, 218.

STRASSBURGER, R. H., and FRENCH, L. A. (1961). *J. Lancet*, **81**, 86.

TALAIRACH, J., and SZIKLA, G. (1965). *Neurochir.*, **11**, 233.

TALAIRACH, J., BANCAUD, J., BONIS, A., SZIKLA, G., and TOURNOUX, P. (1962). *Confin. neurol.*, **22**, 328.

TALAIRACH, J., DAVID, M., TOURNOUX, P., CORREDOR, H., et KVASINA, T. (1957). *Atlas d'anatomie stéréotaxique. Repérage radiologique indirect des noyaux gris contraux, des régions mesencéphalo-sous-optique et hypothalamique de l'homme*. Paris, Masson.

TALAIRACH, J., HECAEN, M., DAVID, M., MONNIER, M., and DE AJURIAGUERRA, J. (1949). *Rev. neurol.*, **81**, 424.

TALAIRACH, J., TOURNOUX, P., and BANCAUD, J. (1960). *Acta neurochir.*, **8**, 153.

TURNER, E. (1963). *J. Neurol. Neurosurg. Psychiat.*, **26**, 285.

TURNER, E. (1966). Personal communication.

VAN BUREN, J. M., and MACCUBBIN, D. A. (1962). *J. Neurosurg.*, **19**, 811.

WALSH, L. (1966). 2nd Symp. Parkinson's Dis. Supplement *J. Neurosurg.*, **24**, 440.

WHITE, J. C., and SWEET, W. H. (1955). *Pain—Its Mechanisms and Neurosurgical Control*. Springfield, Ill. Charles C. Thomas.

CHAPTER 9

ELECTROENCEPHALOGRAPHY IN THE STUDY OF EPILEPSY

M. V. DRIVER

ELECTROENCEPHALOGRAPHY has an established place in the diagnosis of intracranial space occupying lesions and inflammatory, degenerative and vascular lesions of the brain (Hill and Parr, 1963). Its role in the diagnosis of mental diseases is less apparent, though there is no doubt that electrographic methods play, and will continue to play, an important part in experimental psychiatry and psychology. It is in the study of the many and varied manifestations of epilepsy that the EEG has been found of greatest value and a large proportion of the effort of clinical and experimental laboratories is directed to this end. This chapter is concerned with the utilization of electroencephalography in the diagnosis of epilepsy, and in particular of focal epilepsy, and with a discussion of some of the more interesting recent work on epilepsy in childhood, and on spike-wave complexes, the "14 and 6 positive spike phenomenon" and the prognostic value of the EEG in epilepsy.

THE DIAGNOSIS OF EPILEPSY

Epilepsy is a clinical diagnosis, but it is by no means true that all epileptic seizures are sufficiently distinct from non-epileptic phenomena to make the EEG superfluous. The difficulties are well illustrated in an article by Liske and Forster (1964) in which are described 9 cases whose "pseudoseizures" (a term the authors prefer to "hysterical fits") appear quite possibly not to be epileptic. However, one of the patients, though having a normal EEG during a "seizure", did at times have spike-wave bursts in the inter-ictal record. Had several of the patients such bursts it seems unlikely that the attacks would have been labelled "pseudoseizures" and opinions might have changed if all the patients had had EEGs taken during the seizures. One cannot say whether these patients with "pseudoseizures" were epileptic or not, and it seems doubtful whether they can usefully be regarded as a group—the problem is essentially one of diagnosis in the individual and EEG studies are only likely to be of assistance if they are thorough.

Gastaut and Gibson (1960) described methods for the detection and differentiation of fainters and epileptics and concluded that a battery of tests, including occular compression and Valsalva's manœuvre, was of value and they recommended its use in aviation medicine. A reluctance to use such methods in clinical practice is reinforced by the findings of Mewburn and Gibson (1963) that in most positive cases the fainting reaction also occurred when the electrodes were being applied. The effects of emotional stress in patients with definite epilepsy were studied by Small *et al.* (1964), the main finding being that the effect on the EEGs of those with generalized epilepsy, whether major or minor, differed from that on those with focal epilepsy, only the latter being likely to show an "activation" response. Stevens (1962) reported (largely on the same group of patients as Small *et al.*) that patients with generalized epilepsy differed from those with focal epilepsy also in relation to their EEG response to rhythmic stimulation (including light and sound), though in this case it was the "generalized" group which showed the activation response.

It is in cases where the symptoms might also suggest a psychiatric diagnosis that the difficulty more usually arises, and in these the EEG can be of very definite value. Episodic posturing, speechlessness and hallucinatory phenomena are examples. However, just as epilepsy manifests itself clinically as a recurrent and episodic disorder so it does electrically; many minutes or hours of quite normal EEG record may separate the transient phenomena on the presence of which support for the diagnosis of epilepsy depends. A single normal EEG can be of no decisive value in the exclusion of epilepsy, but a few seconds of abnormal activity may well be considered of diagnostic importance.

Many attempts have been made to differentiate between the epileptic and the non-epileptic by measurement of "convulsive threshold". Most have been based on the intravenous injection of leptazol (Metrazol, Cardiazol), the convulsant properties of which were first utilized by von Meduna (1935) in the treatment of schizophrenia. Ziskind *et al.* (1946) suggested that the presence of "larval" attacks in the EEG of epileptics supported the idea that there existed an earlier subclinical indication of neuronal discharge which might be substituted as a measure of a true "convulsive" threshold. They devised an index of excitability based on the first appearance of slow and other abnormal waves in the EEG when a 10 per cent solution of leptazol was injected intravenously at a rate of 1 ml/min. However, experiments showed that in an individual laboratory animal the index could be very variable, even though the electrical convulsive threshold as measured after Putnam and Merritt (1937) was relatively constant, and in human beings no clear line of demarcation could be drawn between the thresholds of epileptic and non-epileptic patients. Subsequent modifications by Cure et al. (1948) and Merlis et al. (1950) were no more successful and it is probable that the diagnostic importance of "threshold" would have ceased to be of interest had it not been for the development by Gastaut (1950) of "photopharmacological activation" in which the slow intravenous injection of leptazol was combined with intermittent photic stimulation. The advantage of this method was that it produced very much more definite end-points short of an active seizure than did the injection alone, and though the various end-points did not have the same significance (Bickford et al. (1952), Ulett et al. (1955)) a patient's threshold appeared to be reasonably constant. Though the method does demonstrate some threshold difference between idio-pathic epileptics and non-epileptics as groups, especially if appropriate allowances are made for cardiac output and other physiological variables (Driver, 1962), variability of EEG response of normal subjects to the injection of convulsants is so great (Sellden, 1964 and Rodin, 1964) that it is of little value in the solution of the in-dividual diagnostic problem and its use for this purpose can rarely, if ever, be justified.

The use of convulsant drugs in the diagnosis of "focal" epilepsy is discussed in a later section.

Two simple methods of "activating" the EEG in the epileptic patient, hyperventilation and photic stimulation are used almost routinely. In the former, the subject is asked to overbreathe at sufficient rate and depth significantly to reduce alveolar carbon dioxide tension. Doubts about the way in which this procedure affects cerebral function have been resolved to some extent by the work of Meyer and Gotoh (1960) in laboratory animals and Gotoh et al. (1965) in human beings. Continuous measurements of gases and electrolytes in arterial and jugular blood, of exhaled carbon dioxide and of respiratory volumes during hyperventilation were made, with simultaneous EEG recordings. It was demonstrated that a reduction of cerebral venous oxygen tension occurred and that this showed a close correlation with the appearance of EEG slowing. The reduction of cerebral venous oxygen tension was mainly due to a decrease in cerebral blood flow, though about a quarter of the reduction could be assigned to the effects of increased blood alkalinity on the stability of oxyhæmoglobin (Bohr effect). Finally, these changes were significantly greater, as is the EEG response to hyperventilation, in the younger age group (below 35) than in the older. An interesting report by Salzman et al. (1963) indicates that the condition induced in an "acute" hyperventilation experiment (e.g. the usual period of 3 minutes in the EEG laboratory) may be quite different from that resulting from long-lasting hyperventilation. Respiratory alkalosis was produced in 13 normal men, aged 20–29 years, and maintained for one hour by voluntary intermittent hyperventilation. Measurements of alveolar CO_2 tension were made (usually reductions to 20 mm Hg, about half normal, were attained) and various estimations were made on arterial blood. It was observed that in only 4 cases did the EEG show prominent high voltage slow activity and this disappeared before the end of the experiment. Salzman et al. suggested that the normal subject can compensate rapidly for hypocapnia and hypoxæmia, and this compensation restores the normal cortical electrical activity. It is impossible to relate these findings adequately to those of Gotoh et al. (1965) since few comparable measurements were made but the hypothesis that anxiety plays a major part in the clinical picture of hyperventilation (as suggested by Salzman et al.) is not unattractive as in the clinical recording situation the effects of hyperventilation are by no means predictable.

The appearance of spike-wave complexes in patients with petit mal epilepsy is often facilitated by this procedure and a definite clinical seizure may be precipitated. The focal spikes of partial epilepsy are less likely to be provoked, though they may sometimes appear during the period of relaxation which follows the resumption of normal breathing, and occasionally a seizure may develop, in which case useful EEG changes may be observed.

Rhythmic photic stimulation (up to about 50 flashes per second) may also elicit typical spike-wave bursts and definite epileptic seizures, though a more common effect is generalized myoclonus during which the subject does not appear to lose consciousness. In the latter state the EEG shows no spikes or complexes of definite cerebral origin, those appearing in the record being muscle artefacts (though recordings from within the brain may disclose a cerebral component also, see Chatrian and Perez-Borja, 1964). This "photomyoclonic response" (Bickford et al. 1952) may be found in apparently normal subjects and in neuropsychiatric patients as well as in epileptics and it is doubtful whether it has any clinical significance. Some children with behaviour disorders show bursts of spike-wave in the

EEG with photic stimulation, though the complexes are usually readily distinguishable from the more typical 3 per second complexes of petit mal and they rarely outlast the stimulus. This phenomenon, and the appearance of other spike-wave phenomena in non-epileptic patients, has been discussed by Rogina and Serafetinides (1962).

In many patients, and particularly those with a long history of epileptic seizures, a single EEG record, which includes periods under hyperventilation and photic stimulation, may be adequate but if there is some doubt concerning the responsible pathology, and especially if the seizures are of recent onset, several records should be taken to establish a more reliable baseline against which any subsequent change can be assessed. Without this precaution any statements regarding "deterioration" or "improvement" are of little or no value.

Television Epilepsy

Photic stimulation has been used as a provocative measure in most of the reported cases of "television epilepsy," almost invariably with success though the conditions of maximum sensitivity are by no means constant. One of the subjects described by Pallis and Louis (1961) had abnormal EEG responses when the eyes were shut, and these responses disappeared on eye opening, whereas two of Mawdsley's (1961) cases had abnormal responses only when the eyes were open and these were inhibited by eye closure. Most of the cases reported by Pantelakis et al. (1962) had abnormal responses whether the eyes were open or shut, though they were more frequently provoked in the latter state, in which, too, the effective range of flash rate was more extended at the lower end (down to 6, in contrast with 16 per second). The last authors were impressed by the ease with which myoclonic jerks and EEG abnormalities were provoked by flicker stimulation in the laboratory and the rarity of the actual "TV" seizures, in view of the large amount of time most of their patients spent watching television. The possible reasons they gave, involving differences in light intensity and on-off contrast, were also considered by Gastaut et al. (1962a) who carried out EEG examinations on similar cases in a television studio, using a television screen (working under normal and abnormal conditions) as the stimulus. None of their patients had spike-wave patterns in the EEG under these circumstances, whereas they invariably did under "stroboscope" stimulation in the EEG laboratory. Seizures occurring before a properly adjusted television set in a not too darkened room are certainly very difficult to explain unless some factor not readily reproduced under experimental conditions (e.g. tiredness, boredom, excitement) is invoked, whereas attacks occurring during adjustments of the screen are more readily explicable. Bickford (1949) showed that "sectored" light stimulation (i.e. movement of alternate light and dark areas across the field of vision) was much more effective in producing paroxysmal EEG discharges in normal subjects than was the more usual "flicker" stimulation, a similar phenomenon being noted by Sherwood (1962) as one of the methods utilized in self-induced epilepsy. He suggested that these subjects had not only a greatly increased sensitivity to light but also hypersensitivity of other parts of the nervous system, for example those subserving gaze. It is possible that patients with television epilepsy have multiple sensitivities, of which the one most readily demonstrated under laboratory conditions is to light. None of Mawdsley's cases had further seizures on being given anticonvulsants and after being told not to look at the television when the screen flickered, but no follow-up was reported on sensitivity to photic stimulation in the laboratory. Personal observation indicates that it need not change, even though the seizures cease.

Sleep

Gibbs et al. (1947) reported that the spike and other phenomena of epilepsy were more commonly seen in the EEG during natural sleep than in the state of wakefulness, since which time a sleep record has been the first choice in further investigations. There appears to be little difference in the efficacy of sleep however it is produced, whether naturally or assisted by such drugs as the barbiturates, methylpentynol (Kennedy and Marley, 1959) etc., given by mouth. The assessment of the sleep record is similar to that of the routine EEG since on the whole similar phenomena appear, though there may be considerable modification of spike-wave bursts (Fig. 18) and even their replacement by multiple spikes (Niedermayer, 1965). The "14 and 6 positive spike" phenomenon of light sleep is discussed in a later section.

In some circumstances, and particularly if sphenoidal electrodes (discussed below) are to be used, sleep may be induced by the slow intravenous injection of thiopentone ($2 \cdot 5$ or 5 per cent solution at 50 mg per minute). This procedure considerably modifies the EEG, very prominent fast (16–24 c/sec) activity appearing in the early stages and continuous spindle activity later. Various slow phenomena also appear but the arousal forms of natural sleep are elicited only with difficulty. If the depth of the narcosis is pushed beyond that at which the corneal reflex disappears (the usual stopping point) a "suppression-burst" type of EEG develops, in which periods of generalized relative flatness of the trace alternate with brief episodes of high voltage slow waves. This method of inducing sleep is valuable in that it not only tends to favour the development of temporal spikes but it can give evidence of local cortical pathology since the fast and other induced activity may be less apparent in the vicinity of a structural lesion. This was noted by Kennedy and Hill (1958) in relation to sphenoidal recordings, particularly in cases of mesial temporal (Ammon's horn) sclerosis. Such a relative reduction of fast activity is not however invariably trustworthy since factors other than pathology, and in particular great frequency of spike production in an area of cortex, can lead to a definite diminution in the ability of that area to participate in the fast thiopentone response. Repeated recordings, to see whether or not the asymmetry is constant, may help to settle this point.

Sleep deprivation may also act as an "activator" of the EEG and may even precipitate an epileptic seizure in susceptible individuals (Bennet, 1963), a phenomenon which seems more likely to be of medico-legal and industrial than clinical importance.

Many other types of simple "activation" have been practised, of which the presentation of the appropriate stimulus in types of "reflex" epilepsy is most likely to be successful (examples are to be found in Poskanzer et al. (1962), Lishman et al. (1962), Goldie and Green (1959). Green (1963) has made a new attempt to popularize the epileptogenic propensities of hypoglycæmia by the intravenous injection of 1 gram of tolbutamide. He stated that it is a safe procedure and that it does not disturb the EEG of normal individuals, but he made no comparison of its effectiveness with sleep and its actual value in diagnosis is not clear. The most interesting aspect is that there was no correlation of effect on the EEG and hypoglycæmia, in view of which Green suggested that different parts of the brain might have different sensitivities to the procedure.

Telemetric devices are finding increasing application in medicine and it is possible that they will occasionally be of value in the primary diagnosis of epilepsy where, as pointed out by Liske et al. (1962), the usual method of recording cannot be used for more than a few hours at a time. However it seems unlikely that the advantages of telemetry can be fully utilized unless some triggering device is available to switch on the EEG recording apparatus at the appropriate time. Alternatively, the EEG could be recorded for hour after hour on magnetic tape, but some recognition system, analogous to a triggering pattern, would be necessary to facilitate subsequent analysis. Such developments require more sophisticated devices than can economically be produced at present.

Sphenoidal Recordings

Electrodes placed on the forehead and scalp are favourably positioned for recording electrical activity of the convexity of the frontal, parietal and occipital lobes and of the superolateral aspect of the temporal lobe. They are much less well placed for recording activity of the inferolateral and inferomesial aspects of the temporal lobe. Since the lesions responsible for temporal lobe epilepsy tend to involve the mesial structures (hippocampus, amygdaloid region) the demonstration of electrical abnormalities in these areas assumes great diagnostic importance.

Knowledge of the types of electrical phenomena met with in the temporal regions of normal subjects is necessary before any assessment of possible "epileptic" activity can be made, but an article by Kooi *et al.* (1964) overemphasizes the difficulties. They examined the EEGs of over 200 normal adults and found that about 25 per cent showed "sharp" waves and about 5 per cent "spikes". However, these phenomena occurred as components of bursts of mixed activity and the frequency of occurrence was approximately the same whether the subjects were drowsy or awake. In both these respects the "abnormalities" differ from those seen in temporal lobe epilepsy, where the sharp waves and spikes exist as quite separate entities and are generally much more common in the drowsy state.

Of the various special electrodes introduced for recording mesial temporal activity only the sphenoidal electrode (Pampiglione and Kerridge 1956) is widely used, though the rigid needle electrode is now usually replaced by a fine insulated silver wire electrode (about 0·15 mm diameter) introduced within a hollow needle which is immediately withdrawn. These electrodes are more comfortable for the patient than the rigid needles and there is no risk of damage to the patient's cheek if he has a seizure. On the other hand, the wires are somewhat more difficult to introduce and are more prone to lead to artefacts than the needles.

Rovit *et al.* (1961a) modified the procedure by using twin electrodes on each side, one directed anteriorly to the lateral pterygopalatine fossa and the other posteriorly to the posterior edge of the foramen ovale (the usual position of the single electrode is about half-way between these sites). They also inserted a nasopharyngeal electrode.

In their "unilateral" temporal cases roughly one third had adequately localizable foci at the scalp electrodes, a further third at the pharyngeal electrode and the remainder only at a sphenoidal. In the "bilateral" temporal cases about a quarter were adequately assessed with the scalp electrodes and another quarter with the pharyngeal, the remainder needing the sphenoidals. The main conclusion—which confirms the experience of others—was that such a technique was of particular value in determining the presence or absence of bilaterality of abnormality (Fig. 17). The fact that on occasion spikes can appear at only one of the twin electrodes appears to make impossible an

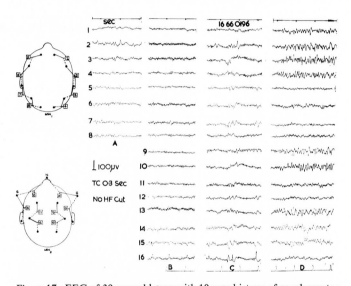

Figure 17. EEG of 30 year old man with 10 year history of psychomotor seizures. *A*. Patient awake: sharp waves of probable right anterior temporal origin (channel 2). *B*. Patient alerted by insertion of sphenoidal electrodes: the sharp waves in *A* are no longer present but frequent sharp waves appear as a left sphenoidal focus (channels 15, 16). These are seen only with difficulty from the scalp (channels 5, 6, 7) but are probably responsible for the indistinct irregularities of the left temporal scalp in *A*. *C*. Light sleep during slow intravenous injection of thiopentone: right and left temporal sharp waves appear, independent in time and not in homologous areas. *D*. Immediately before waking up: a possible 'seizure' discharge affecting the right sylvian-temporal cortex. Radiology demonstrated a filling defect of the right temporal horn of the lateral ventricle and subsequent operation disclosed a small mass (a hamartoma, possibly ectopic grey matter) occluding the horn.

assumption of strictly unilateral involvement, though this is unlikely to lead to practical difficulties.

In laboratories undertaking intensive investigations of temporal lobe epilepsy as a prelude to assessment for surgical operation two or more sphenoidal recordings may be carried out, in one of which sleep will be induced slowly by oral ingestion of quinalbarbitone sodium (Seconal) or a similar drug, and in the others more rapidly by the intravenous injection of thiopentone as described above. Various other drugs including chlorpromazine (Lyberi and Last, 1956), imipramine (Kiloh *et al.*, 1966) and amitriptylene (Davison, 1965) have been given intravenously as EEG "activators" in such investigations but it is doubtful whether they offer advantage over the barbiturates in any respect. They have the defect of not inducing fast activity, asymmetry of which can be a useful lateralizing feature.

Recording during thiopentone induced narcosis in temporal lobe epilepsy so commonly demonstrates focal spikes, sharp waves or spike-slow complexes at a sphenoidal or other temporal electrode that their failure to appear in one or two repeated records raises serious doubts about the original diagnosis. Quite the opposite is true with some other common sites of epileptogenic lesions, and in particular the sensorimotor cortex, where repeated interictal EEG recordings may show no abnormality, whether the patient is asleep or awake. In such cases focal spikes may eventually appear if leptazol or bemegride is injected slowly intravenously.

FURTHER INVESTIGATIONS

If a neurosurgical operation for the relief of epilepsy is contemplated the degree to which EEG investigation should be carried out depends solely on the requirements of the case. In most instances more elaborate techniques than the sleep record with or without sphenoidal electrodes are not called for. This is probably almost always so when EEG abnormalities have been strictly unilateral and limited in distribution. It is sometimes so even though there are bilateral temporal spike foci, provided one side shows additional gross electrical abnormality or other evidence of lateralization is available (e.g. radiological) or, and this is certainly less reliable, one side consistently and under all circumstances shows a far more frequently discharging spike focus than the other. However, many patients with epilepsy severe enough to warrant neurosurgery have more equal bilateral abnormalities in the EEG and the side significantly involved (if such there be) in the seizures is apparent neither in routine and sleep recordings nor from clinical, radiological etc., findings. The two situations in which this is likely to be met with are psychomotor epilepsy with asynchronous bilateral temporal spike foci and "secondary subcortical epilepsy" (Penfield and Jasper, 1954) in which widespread and synchronous bilateral spike-wave complexes appear in the EEG.

It is appropriate at this point to discuss some recent findings in experimental epilepsy as they have contributed to, though not provided the sole basis for, the development of the EEG techniques used in the more difficult diagnostic problems.

(i) *Mirror Foci*

An experimental lesion in the cortex of one hemisphere may result, not only in a local spike focus, but also in a "mirror" focus in the homologous area of the other hemisphere (Morrell 1959, 1960). To begin with, the spikes of the mirror focus appear to represent a disturbance transmitted directly from the primary lesion since they follow the primary spikes after an interval of a few milliseconds and are abolished by section of the corpus callosum. Early removal of the lesion leads to the disappearance of both the primary and the transmitted mirror spikes. If the lesion is not removed at this stage spikes may ultimately appear in the contralateral hemisphere independently in time of the ipsilateral spikes and subsequent removal of the lesion or section of the corpus callosum becomes less effective. Lesions of the amygdaloid nucleus and hippocampus in cats may also lead to the production of bilateral independent spike foci, and excision of the primary lesion or section of the corpus callosum and other commissures does not necessarily lead to disappearance of the contralateral spikes (Gastaut and Fischer-Williams 1959; Guerrero-Figueroa *et al.* (1964)). It is commonly supposed that in such cases the contralateral structures have acquired an epileptogenic potential through being "bombarded" by discharges from the vicinity of the lesion, and that the excitability of the area homologous to the lesion may ultimately become as great as, or even greater than, that of the primary area. Morrell (1960) stated that the contralateral alterations in function manifest in the mirror focus ultimately become permanently fixed and independent of the system responsible for their establishment. He also demonstrated chemical changes in the cells of the mirror focus which also persisted after excision of the primary lesion. However, recent studies with microelectrodes (Ajmone-Marsan, 1963) show what seem to be important differences between the primary and the transmitted foci: the latter appear against a background of much less intense neuronal discharge, both in terms of the number of units activated and in the frequency of spike occurrence.

This finding suggests that the contralateral mirror discharge is not a manifestation of a potentially "epileptogenic" process.

The confirmation that similar mirror foci with similar properties could be artificially produced in the temporal lobes of human beings would not necessarily be of decisive importance since it is unlikely that the pathology, time course, spatial extent and so on of the "natural" epileptogenic lesion could be produced. However, a number of relevant observations can be made on EEG findings in cases of temporal lobe epilepsy:

1. It is not uncommon, even with a history of many years, to find spikes entirely confined to one side.

2. When spike foci occur bilaterally they rarely show any obvious time relationship however young the patient or (apparently) recent the lesion, nor need they appear in precisely homologous areas.

3. Unilateral temporal lobectomy may result in eventual disappearance of apparently independent spike foci from both sides.

4. Unilateral anterior temporal spike foci and psychomotor seizures may result from posterior temporal lesions and both may disappear following local removal of the lesion (Falconer *et al.*, 1962).

5. Patients may show what is probably a "projected" disturbance, for example spike and wave, when adolescent but exclusively anterior temporal spike foci when adult.

It can be concluded that in temporal lobe epilepsy several directions of transmission from the area of the lesion are possible, one of which may resemble the "mirror" variety of experimental work. The failure of long-standing cases to show bilateral spikes in the EEG suggests that transmission outside one temporal lobe is not invariable though Ajmone-Marsan's observations on the dissimilarity between neuronal events in the region of the primary and mirror foci allows of the speculation that given the time scale of development of human epilepsy such phenomena may in some circumstances be temporary.

Perhaps the most important observation is that many patients with bilateral temporal spikes in the EEG get considerable or complete relief from seizures following a unilateral temporal lobectomy. Whatever the phenomena responsible for the bilateral EEG abnormalities, one temporal lobe in such cases appears to have a sufficient degree of dominance in the initiation or elaboration of the seizures to make its identification a valid diagnostic procedure.

(ii) *Secondary Subcortical Epilepsy*

A variety of generalized epilepsy is occasionally met with in cases having a demonstrable localized cerebral pathology (Tükel and

Jasper, 1952) and in particular with cicatrizant lesions (e.g. chronic abscesses) of the orbital and mesial regions of the frontal lobe. The EEG may be indistinguishable from that commonly seen in idiopathic minor epilepsy, showing regularly repetitive spike-wave complexes, but more usually some irregularity of frequency, form or distribution is apparent (Fig. 18). The interictal EEG may also show features not commonly seen in idiopathic epilepsy, such as localized slow activity, but a definite and constant spike focus is relatively uncommon. It is assumed that though the epilepsy presumably relates to dysfunction brought about by the presence of the lesion (surgical removal of which can result in abatement of the

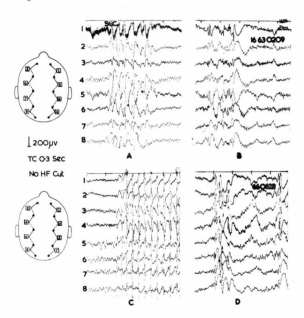

Figure 18. EEGs of 15 year old girl (*A* and *B*) with daily minor 'absence' seizures and monthly major convulsive seizures from the age of 11 (previous history of left mastoid infection with cerebral abscess at 7) and of 15 year old boy (*C* and *D*) with daily minor 'absence' seizures, no major convulsive seizures and no relevant antecedents. The spike-wave complexes are less well formed and less regularly repetitive in *A* than in *C* (patients awake). The complexes of the sleeping state (*B* and *D*) are less readily distinguishable. At operation the girl was found to have a chronic abscess in the left orbitomesial frontal region, following resection of which the fits ceased altogether and the spike-wave complexes no longer appeared in the EEG (2-year follow-up).

seizures and disappearance of the spike-wave phenomenon) the initial epileptic process utilizes the same pathways as does idiopathic epilepsy.

This variety of seizures can be considered to occupy a broad intermediate position between "idiopathic" or "centrencephalic" (Penfield and Jasper, 1954) epilepsy in which, though the initiating process may not itself be in the upper brain stem (Williams, 1965), it is not dependent on a definite cortical lesion, and a focal or partial epilepsy with secondary generalization (Gastaut, 1964) in which signs of cortical involvement (e.g. sensorimotor phenomena) precede the loss of consciousness. Though these seizure types appear to form a continuum with no very definite clinical or electrographic demarcation, it is useful to recognize a group in which the objective and subjective phenomena of the attack are not exactly those of a "typical" generalized seizure and the spike-wave or other complexes of the EEG do not have the "typical" regularity and frequency seen in petit mal.

As noted above, experimental cortical and hippocampal lesions usually lead to the production of mirror foci, and even in preparations in which lesions of the intralaminar thalamic nuclei and the reticular formation lead to the development of spike-wave complexes similar lesions in the cortex do not (see discussion of the spike-wave phenomenon below). On the other hand the experiments reported by Wilder and Schmidt (1965) showed that in monkeys with chronic neocortical foci spread of the discharges during an actual seizure involved the basal nuclei, reticular formation and the diffuse thalamic projection nuclei with the development of spike-wave complexes. However, as Kennedy (1959) observed, small lesions in epileptic patients, even if in the effective areas (Tükel and Jasper, 1952), do not lead to spike-wave formation in the EEG and it seems probable that extensive lesions involving both cortex and subcortex are necessary, with dysfunction of both ends of the thalamocortical systems.

The Drug-induced Seizure

Focal epileptic seizures, and particularly those of temporal lobe origin, are frequently associated with a localized or at least a lateralized "discharge" in the EEG. This discharge may take the form of a series of spike-sharp complexes, of spikes, of regular rhythmic waves or of mixed phenomena. The components characteristically change in frequency and voltage as the attack continues, a progression from a low voltage fast (say 7–14/sec) to a higher voltage slow (say 3/sec) pattern being not uncommon. Immediately preceding the discharge there may be a period (usually up to 5 seconds or so) during which is seen a flattening of the EEG in the area in which the discharge will develop, other areas continuing to show the pre-ictal pattern. Since such phenomena are commonly seen in the vicinity of the experimental epileptogenic lesion and can be produced by local electrical stimulation of the human brain, it is assumed that when they occur spontaneously they do so in the area in which the seizure is developing. Identification of such phenomena can therefore be of great importance in otherwise obscure cases of epilepsy, and in particular in those with multifocal interictal spikes in which, though no different significance can be attached to the spikes on one side or in one location than to those elsewhere, the general consistency of the habitual attacks (where such is indeed the case) is indicative of a probable uniqueness of origin and spread.

However, even though a period is chosen when the patient appears most liable to have a seizure, or though some supposedly adequate stimulus is given, and though the patient's anticonvulsant drugs map be withdrawn, no seizure may occur during the time available for EEG recording. In such circumstances a seizure may be induced by injection of a convulsant drug, and provided the patient's habitual seizure is in fact provoked the conclusions drawn are valid.

To what extent is the induced fit a true reproduction of those occurring spontaneously? Injection of sufficient of a convulsant drug will lead to the development of an epileptic seizure in a normal healthy subject, but the seizure will be generalized from the beginning. It will, in fact, be identical with the "major" tonic-clonic seizure. A similar seizure will be induced, though perhaps more readily, in a patient whose spontaneous attacks are of this type. Quite different seizures may follow the injection in patients with focal epilepsy and in some patients who have cerebral lesions (e.g. tumours) but no spontaneous epileptic attacks. In focal epileptics the seizures show features reported in the habitual attack and perhaps others which, though not reported as a part of the spontaneous attack pattern, relate to dysfunction of the diseased part of the brain or of an area in some way related to it. For example, the assumption of a tonic posture of one arm, the elbow being flexed and the shoulder abducted and externally rotated, is common during the drug in-duced psychomotor attack, though it is less often reported in the spontaneous seizures. This posture can be related to disturbed func-tion of the contralateral temporal and supplementary motor areas (Ajmone-Marsan and Ralston, 1957). The drug-induced focal seizure may proceed more commonly, and more quickly, to a generalized convulsive seizure than does the habitual, but it rarely does so unless the patient has, or has had, some spontaneous generalized seizures. It appears probable that differences between drug-induced and spontaneous seizures are not expressions of different origins within the brain but of different pathways of spread. The spontaneous seizure develops against a background of what is for the patient normal cerebral activity, the induced seizure develops in the most sensitive area of a brain brought near functional disintegration by the convulsant drug. It is contended that valid conclusions can be drawn from the induced fit pattern and from the simultaneous EEG (Fig. 19) (see also Goldensohn, 1962).

The seizure is generally induced by the slow intravenous injection of leptazol (Ajmone-Marsan and Ralston, 1957; Driver *et al.*, 1964), though bemegride is equally effective (Sellden, 1964) and some have used an inhalent convulsant "Indoklon" (discussed in Symposium

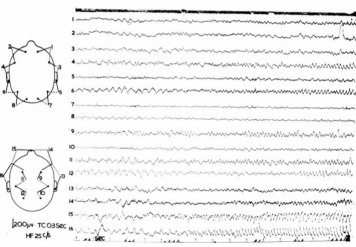

Figure 19. Leptazol induced psychomotor seizure: the pre-ictal pattern is of predominantly left hemisphere slow activity (channels 4, 6, 11, 12, 15, 16), which is replaced when the seizure starts by a rhythmic high voltage "ictal" sharp wave discharge which is seen most prominently at the left sphenoidal electrode (channels 15 and 16). The seizure would appear to be of left cerebral hemisphere and probably temporal origin. No confirmatory evidence was obtained by other means and, the resting and sleeping EEG showing bilateral and multifocal spikes, no operative treatment was attempted.

on Indoklon, 1962, see also Chatrian and Petersen, 1960). The reader is referred to Sellden (*loc. cit.*) for a comprehensive discussion of the effects of convulsant drugs on the EEG of the normal human subject. The procedure is photographed, preferably by a cine camera with a large film magazine and running at a reduced speed (8 frames per second is adequate). The recent availability of simple television cameras and videorecording systems promises to make the visual recording easier and less expensive than it has been. The filmed phenomena may provide some confirmation of lateralization, and may in fact be the sole lateralizing evidence if the ictal EEG is, as sometimes happens, lost in muscle and movement artefacts. Clinical examination of the patient during and after the seizure may also disclose signs of lateralizing or localizing importance (e.g. dysphasia, hemianopia, hemiparesis, etc.).

Though of great value in the lateralization of the seizure in cases of known epilepsy (Ajmone-Marsan and Ralston, 1957; Ajmone-Marsan and Abraham, 1960; Kennedy and Driver, 1962, Rodin, 1964, Rodin *et al.*, 1964) the technique has little value, and if used should be interpreted with great caution, in cases where there is doubt that the patient's symptoms are in fact epileptic and where all previous studies have had negative results. The symptoms (e.g. sudden attacks of rage and violence) may in fact be exactly reproduced during the slow intravenous injection of leptazol but very rarely are they accompanied by significant EEG changes or by lateralized phenomena, nor do they develop into a generalized convulsive seizure. The whole procedure can be a very trying one for the patient and it is not surprising that in some circumstances the stress is as active a provoker of a psychoneurotic reaction in a susceptible person as is the leptazol itself of a true seizure in a patient with epilepsy.

Multiple Intracranial Electrodes

It is readily demonstrable that the conventional scalp EEG gives a very limited view of changes in electrical potential occurring within the brain. The potential averaging effect of the extracerebral tissues and of the electrodes themselves results in marked attenuation of spatially limited potential changes so that though low voltage but widespread rhythmic changes can be recorded in the EEG, relatively high voltage but very localized changes cannot be distinguished from other activity. In certain circumstances, for example with evoked cortical responses to sensory stimulation, and with suitable magnetic tape recordings showing some obvious phenomenon which can be used as a "triggering" signal, a computer can be used to extract such apparently lost potentials from the more random activity. However, more generally the resolution of the conventional ink-writing oscillographs cannot significantly be bettered and a more detailed appreciation of intracerebral potential changes can only be obtained by the use of intracranial electrodes.

The first detailed reports on the use of chronically implanted electrodes in human beings and the techniques employed appeared some years ago (Delgado, 1952; Mayo Symposium, 1953), more recent publications being Chatrian *et al.* (1959a and b), Llewellyn and Heath (1962), Fischer-Williams and Cooper (1963) and Crandall

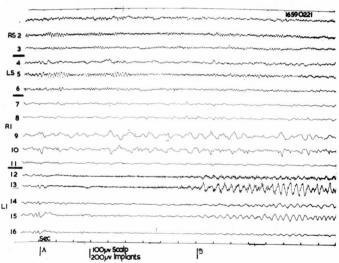

Figure 20. Leptazol induced seizure: RS (channels 1–3) and LS (channels 4–6) are right and left scalp EEG of the temporal regions. RI (channels 7–11) and LI (channels 12–16) are multiple implanted electrodes in the right and left temporal lobes (6-contact wire electrodes, 1 cm separation; consecutive bipolar linkages; channels 7 and 12 relate to region of amygdaloid nuclei, 11 and 16 to cortex of lateral aspect of temporal lobe). At *A* (start of "electrical seizure") the activity of LI decreases in amplitude and fast activity appears in the deeper regions. At *B* more widespread left temporal slow activity develops. These changes do not involve the conventional scalp EEG (LS). Clinical seizure activity (a psychomotor attack) began only some 10 sec. following the end of this excerpt. The patient had a small glial hamartoma of the amygdala, with Ammon's horn sclerosis.

et al. (1963), while Bates (1961) and several other authors contribute to a comprehensive discussion on all aspects of the subject. On the whole, experience has shown that such electrodes are much more rarely of use than might be supposed. In the circumstances of the main indication for their use, that is in the presence of bilateral or multiple hemispheric spike or other foci, it is to be expected that the intracerebral electrical phenomena recorded will be anything but simple. Though a distinction between "significant" and "non-significant" spikes has been made by Ralston (1958) on the basis of the presence of an "afterdischarge" with the former, this has not been adequately confirmed in human epilepsy, and in practice such a distinction is impossible. The significance of slow activity and apparent deficiencies of "normal" activity as recorded from deeply implanted electrodes is too difficult to assess to be acceptable as evidence of localization. It may occasionally be possible to reproduce the patient's aura or even to provoke a seizure of the habitual pattern by electrical stimulation of one of the electrodes, in which case an important inference can be drawn. A more reliable method of inducing seizure phenomena is the intravenous injection of a convulsant drug (as described above), which may lead to a very clear electrographic localization (Fig. 20). However, these electrodes record only from a very limited volume of brain and it is quite possible for the patient clearly to be having a focal epileptic seizure with no accompanying change in the activity recorded by the depth electrodes. Crandall *et al.* (1963) have reported optimistically on the use of implanted electrodes in certain cases of temporal lobe epilepsy and it is possible that their careful stereotactic technique is a real step forward.

Intracarotid Injection Techniques

The injection of amylobarbitone into the carotid arteries of man was first utilized by Wada (1949) for lateralization of cerebral dominance for speech function. Subsequent publications (Wada and Rasmussen, 1960; Serafetinides *et al.*, 1965a) have confirmed the general validity of the procedure. Preliminary contrast angiography may demonstrate bilateral filling of the anterior cerebral arteries but it is considered unlikely that where the arterial circle is symmetrical the amylobarbitone, provided it is injected slowly, crosses to the contralateral circulation in significant amount.

Serafetinides *et al.* (1965b) distinguished three patterns of EEG change following injection: firstly, the very rapid appearance of high voltage rhythmic slow waves; secondly, the very gradual appearance of low voltage fast or 8–13 c/sec or intermediate slow activity and, thirdly, a composite pattern beginning as the gradual type but later developing into a high voltage slow picture of the first type. These changes were all ipsilateral to the injection and appeared to be dependent on the rate of injection rather than on the amount of amylobarbitone injected. Since both epileptic and non-epileptic patients have similar patterns in this respect it seems likely that these would also be the responses of normal brain. The presence of a gross structural lesion on one side may prolong the response on that side very considerably.

The effects of intracarotid injections of up to about 200 mg of sodium amylobarbitone are of brief duration if simple clinical or EEG criteria are used, the pre-injection state returning in almost all cases in about ten minutes (see also Bladin, 1963). An interval of 30 minutes between the injections on the two sides is considered sufficient to allow valid comparison of effects but detailed psychological testing and more sophisticated EEG techniques (e.g. continuous display of rates of change in amount of fast activity) would be necessary to confirm whether or not this is so. That a residuum of effect is still present after 30 minutes is believed by Gloor *et al.* (1964) possibly to account for the mild clinical response to the subsequent intracarotid injection of leptazol (see below).

The use of this technique in the diagnosis of epilepsy depends on the facts that profound functional change can be induced in one cerebral hemisphere at a time, and that the internal carotid artery does not distribute the amylobarbitone to a sufficiently large part of the upper brain stem and diencephalon to induce more generalized disturbances.

Morrell (1960) demonstrated in the experimental animal (cat) that responses to the intracarotid injection of amylobarbitone were variable, whether the injection was given into the side of the lesion or into that with the secondary mirror focus. For example, primary side injection might be followed by a prolonged period of "suppression" of spikes on both sides, or by a brief period of bilateral suppression succeeded by augmentation of spiking on the mirror side alone or both sides. However, when the effects of subsequent removal of the primary lesion were known, it became apparent that there was a high positive correlation between suppression of the secondary spikes with primary side injections and ultimate disappearance of these spikes following the operation. The effects of injections of amylobarbitone into the secondary hemisphere showed no relation to the outcome of surgery.

Coceani *et al.* (1966) carried out similar experiments with penicillin induced lesions in monkeys and showed that it was possible for an injection on one side to suppress not only the ipsilateral primary spikes and the contralateral mirror spikes secondary to it, but also the ipsilateral spikes secondary to a contralateral primary focus, the latter itself being unaffected. However, such experiments did not always give consistent results, in one instance an anomaly of blood supply being held responsible. Coceani *et al.* pointed out that differing pressures of injection might give questionable results, especially in rabbits, a point which had been insufficiently appreciated in previous experimental work. That a similar possibility exists with human subjects is suggested by the data published by Serafetinides *et al.* (1965a) where in a total of 24 angiograms there were 14 showing filling of the major vessels confined to the anterior and middle cerebral arteries and 10 showing additional filling of the posterior communicating and posterior cerebral arteries. In 5 cases the filled vessels differed on the two sides and in 9 both anterior cerebral arteries filled with an injection on one side though not with one on the other.

Exactly analogous trials of suppression of foci in human beings would be extremely difficult as the experimental animals were essentially acute preparations. If in fact some patients have independent bilateral foci, one side having been originally "primary" and the other side "secondary," their tests might correspond to part of Morrell's (1960) experiment, i.e. the removal of lesions which had been present the longest time (21–90 days). In these animals neither contralateral amylobarbitone nor removal of the lesion commonly resulted in the disappearance of the secondary spikes, though in the few cases which did show disappearance of spikes following resection injection of amylobarbitone was in fact invariably effective.

Rovit *et al.* (1961b) used the technique in two patients who had "EEG changes indicating the presence of independent bitemporal cortical epileptogenic activity." Each had the injection on only one side, with similar effects: suppression of the focal abnormality ipsilaterally with no change contralaterally. This resembled their findings in three patients with unilateral spike foci, in which injection on the side of the focus suppressed the spikes whereas injection on the other side (done in only two cases) had no effect. Tengesdal (1963) reported similar results with unilateral foci. Perez-Borja and Rivers (1963) carried out the test in one patient with bilateral independent temporal lobe foci and in one with a unilateral temporal lobe focus, finding that injection into one side could produce either suppression of an ipsilateral focus or activation of the ipsilateral or of the contralateral focus. No very definite conclusion can be drawn from these results which confirm that in the study of epilepsy hypotheses based on animal experiments can be very difficult to test in the human subject.

The technique has also been used in the study of patients with "primary bilateral synchrony" (i.e. having a regular spike-wave EEG pattern and petit mal seizures) and "secondary bilateral synchrony" (i.e. having a possibly less regular spike-wave pattern with atypical seizures). This latter phenomenon has been discussed above and also, with reference to the present discussion, by Rovit *et al.* (1961b).

Rovit *et al.* gave bilateral intracarotid injections of sodium amylobarbitone to four patients with clinical and EEG patterns characteristic of petit mal epilepsy (all had major convulsive seizures also) with common findings irrespective of the side of injection. On the side of the injection there was no change in frequency of spike and wave bursts, though the spike component tended to decrease in amplitude, and there was occasionally a provocation of spike-wave activity bilaterally, apart from which no contralateral change occurred. The procedure was repeated in five patients with what was assumed, on the basis of EEG and clinical deviations from the "primary" pattern, to be "secondary bilateral synchrony." In these patients injection into one hemisphere, that assumed to contain the responsible focus, led to elimination of spike-wave activity bilaterally whereas injection into the other hemisphere led to findings resembling those in true petit mal, i.e. no decrease in the frequency of paroxysmal bursts but some decrease in spike amplitude ipsilaterally and a tendency to provoke bilateral discharges. Perez-Borja and Rivers (1963) also tested a case of "secondary bilateral synchrony" by this technique and concluded that the results were essentially in accord with those of Rovit *et al.*

One of the difficulties in interpretation of the results of this test is that the injections can rarely be given actually during the course of a burst of spike-wave activity, and assessment of "suppression" generally depends on comparison of the number and character of the complexes in a 10–15 minute period after the injection with a similar period before. Rovit *et al.* attempted to "activate" the record before the test by reduction of anticonvulsant medication, by intra-muscular injection of chlorpromazine and, in three patients, by the parenteral injection of leptazol. Even so, in only 3 instances out of a total of 35 injections was an actual electroencephalographic and minor clinical seizure in progress at the time. Perez-Borja and Rivers gave their injections during hyperventilation induced seizures, though their illustrations of the EEGs at the time do not appear to be exactly comparable.

Intracarotid injections of leptazol have been given by Gloor *et al.* (1964) with the object of comparing the ease of provocation of electroencephalographic or clinical manifestations of a seizure between one cerebral hemisphere and the other. They tested nine patients whose previous EEGs had suggested the possibility of a secondary bilateral synchrony, and in each the leptazol injections followed the sodium amylobarbitone test which was as described above. In two cases, where the latter suggested that the epilepsy was primary ("centrencephalic"), the amounts of leptazol needed to cause sustained bilateral spike-wave bursts were very similar on the two sides (20 to 25 mg), and in three, where the amylobarbitone test suggested secondary epilepsy, the amounts of leptazol needed to give the same response differed considerably on the two sides (12·5 to 25 mg on one side, 50 to 150 on the other—and that not always sufficient). The other cases, however, gave contrary results: two whose amylobarbitone test suggested "centrencephalic" epilepsy had large differences in amounts of leptazol (one side approximately twice the other) and two whose amylobarbitone test suggested secondary bilateral synchrony had very similar "thresholds" to leptazol. Evaluation of these results is impossible in the absence of definite knowledge of the pathological lesions, where such exist, and until this is available it would appear unreasonable to conclude that the findings in one test go far to support or refute those of the other.

Personal experience with these tests confirms that interpretation of the results is not easy. This may be because few patients in this category have in fact a single epileptogenic lesion confined to part of one cerebral hemisphere. There is also the problem in the individual patient of deciding whether or not the total situation is precisely the same at the time of the second injection as it was for the first. Even so, if a surgical operation is to have a rational basis, the problem of lateralization must be solved and there appear to be reasonable grounds for the belief that in some cases, though possibly few, these techniques may give sufficient support to one possibility or another to enable a decision to be made.

Electrocorticography

The term *electrocorticography*, as commonly used, includes recordings, not only from electrodes placed on the surface of the cerebral cortex as made accessible by a craniotomy, but also from needle or flexible wire electrodes inserted into other structures such as the white matter, the amygdaloid nucleus, the lateral ventricle etc., at the same time. The major difficulty of electrocorticography is at once obvious: a very limited view of the brain is available and no exact comparison can be made between the activity of the two sides. If spikes appear with high frequency in channels recording from the surface of the exposed temporal lobe when pre-operative EEG records have demonstrated bilateral firing no new conclusion can be drawn from this fact alone and there is no confirmation that the responsible lesion is on that side. Various attempts have been made to differentiate between spikes in the vicinity of an actual lesion and "transmitted" or "conducted" spikes which might show as foci in quite normal cortex at a distance from the lesion. Penfield and Jasper (1954) described cortical spikes found in the vicinity of an epileptogenic lesion as similar in every respect to the spikes produced by local application of strychnine to normal cortex, whereas transmitted spikes were usually of lower voltage and of longer duration. However, this is a distinction difficult or impossible to make in practice.

Ralston (1958) studied the high voltage spikes in the vicinity of penicillin lesions of the cortex of cats and monkeys and observed that superimposed on the relatively long duration positive phase which followed the more rapid initial negative deflexion there was occasionally a low voltage 20–40 c/s rhythm or "afterdischarge." These afterdischarges might be very brief; they might be prolonged slightly to give a "larval seizure," or they might continue for a long period as an electrographic seizure, possibly accompanied by objective seizure phenomena in the animal. During prolonged periods of afterdischarge the focal spikes would be absent, as they commonly are in many spontaneously occurring seizures in the human subject. Ralston concluded that the rapid rhythmical afterdischarge was in the majority of cases the precursor of the actual seizure activity. The "projected" spikes at a distance from the lesion showed no afterdischarge phenomena, nor did they appear to develop into actual seizure activity. Identification of a spike with afterdischarge could thus be considered equivalent to identification of the actual lesion. A subsequent publication (Ralston and Papatheodorou, 1960) described the findings at operation in three patients with epilepsy, one of whom showed such afterdischarges spontaneously. Personal observation of this phenomenon in operations for relief of temporal lobe epilepsy has not confirmed that the afterdischarge is a very accurate pointer to the site of maximum pathological damage. However, human epileptogenic lesions may well be far more wide-

spread and complex than pencillin-induced foci in animals, and even
if chronic partial neuronal isolation is a basic factor in the development of "epileptic" activity in the cortex (Echlin and Battista, 1963)
the "isolation" may be too patchy to allow of easy analysis (Fig. 21).

Some other index of abnormal cortical function is necessary, and
Penfield and Jasper (1954) considered a spike focus of definite significance only if it were associated with an objective lesion of the cortex
or with abnormal background activity, by which they meant the

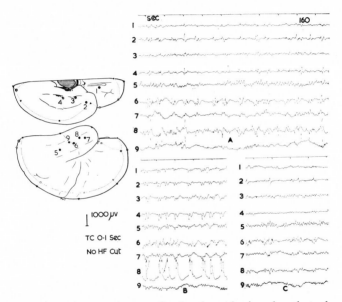

Figure 21. Electrocorticogram (local scalp analgesia only; electrodes
1–7 on cortical surface, 8 and 9 in area of amygdala and hippocampus
respectively; average reference recording, 7 other electrodes not included in these excerpts from 16 channel record). *A* shows high voltage
amygdalar spikes (8) with varying amplitude and time relationship to
surface spikes (2, 4, 6). Electrode 6 (on middle temporal gyrus) shows
fast spike activity having some similarity with "after-discharge"
spikes and the "isolation" phenomenon of experimental epilepsy
(see text). *B* demonstrates the after-discharge following electrical stimulation of the amygdala (8). Though the patient experienced one of his
usual seizures there is no obvious involvement of electrode 6, nor is 6
affected during the period of amygdalar spike absence following the
seizure (*C*). Histologically the resected temporal lobe showed a small
lesion of the amygdala, possibly a glial hamartoma, with normal cortex
in all areas.

absence of the normal cortical rhythms or the presence of irregular slow waves. In this case the spike focus loses all significance except as a guide to an area of cortex which, on close inspection, may appear to have an abnormal configuration or structure, or which may be the seat of other abnormal electrical activity (Fig. 22). Such electro-corticographic evidence is of greatest value during operations for sensorimotor epilepsy when lateralization may be obvious from the seizure pattern but exact localization is uncertain. In addition, the electrocorticographic pattern may be altered in a significant way by the intravenous injection of thiopentone (to increase the amount of fast activity in normal areas of cortex) or of leptazol (to "activate" the spike focus when it is not previously apparent). These procedures are most valuable when the patient is not anæsthetized.

It has been observed that the only definite spike focus may be at a considerable distance from a demonstrable lesion which is itself apparently "silent" in regard to epileptic activity. In addition, the

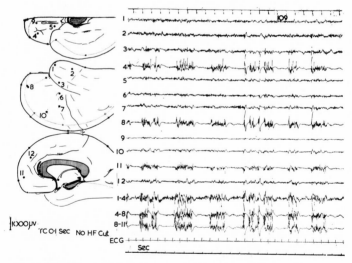

Figure 22. Electrocorticogram, all electrodes on cortical surface. The previous recording (patient awake) had shown multifocal frontal spikes. Following intravenous injection of thiopentone a prominent "isolation" phenomenon ("suppression-burst") appeared at electrodes 4, 8 and 11. The responsible pathology was tuberose sclerosis involving the frontal pole. The more widespread synchrony of the abnormality here in comparison with that localized to electrode 6 in fig. 5 possibly indicates a more intense "isolation" and therefore a more adjacent lesion.

seizure pattern itself may appear more appropriately to be assigned to dysfunction of the area in which the spikes occur. In such cases removal of the lesion rather than the area of electrical abnormality (and apparent origin of the seizures) has had a successful outcome (Falconer et al., 1962).

Appropriate electrical stimulation of the brain may give rise to sensations and to movements, but caution must be used in their interpretation if similar phenomena are part of the spontaneous epileptic attack. Electrical stimulation may also result in a change in the electrical activity of nearby cortex and a true afterdischarge may appear and outlast the stimulus by many seconds. Such afterdischarges can develop in quite normal cortex and are generally not contributory to the actual problem. However, the spatial distribution of the afterdischarge accompanying an electrically induced seizure of the patient's habitual type may be of significance.

It has been observed that removal of all "spiking" cortex is not necessary for a good surgical result (see Magnus et al., 1962) but some attempt at prognosis has been made on the basis of the degree to which this has been done. Jasper et al. (1961) rated all patients post-operatively into one of four categories ranging from no improvement to complete freedom from seizures. They also rated the post-resection electrocorticogram into four categories from persistence of important spike abnormality to complete removal of all areas showing such spikes. The ratings were sufficiently highly correlated to indicate that the method was of definite value in assessing the degree of success of the operation. Goldensohn (1962) however, felt that in his subjects (all cases of temporal lobe epilepsy whereas those of Jasper et al. probably included extra-temporal focal epileptics also) the presence of post-resection spikes in the electrocorticogram had no relation to the ultimate outcome. Silfvenius et al. (1964) came to a similar conclusion with respect to spikes recorded in the insula during operations for temporal lobe epilepsy: the ultimate results were similar whether the affected areas were removed or not.

Conclusion

Many electrographic aids to the diagnosis of epilepsy are now available, some well tried and some of as yet unproven value. Several of the methods need far greater resources than are commonly found in departments of electroencephalography but all should be possible in those centres where epilepsy is treated by neurosurgery. To modify a statement by Green and Scheetz (1964): if EEG localization is not, or cannot, be made by one or other of these methods the chances of successful surgery are slender.

EEG AND EPILEPSY IN CHILDHOOD

Recent interest in the study of the relation between clinical and electrographic aspects of epilepsy in childhood stems largely from the reports of Gibbs and Gibbs (1952) on "hypsarrhythmia" and infantile spasms and of Gastaut et al. (1957) on "hemiconvulsive" seizures. Passouant and Cadilhac (1962) published a comprehensive study of seizure types and associated EEGs met with in children, with particular reference to changes with age. They found that in the newborn seizures generally showed EEG evidence of focal origin, though sometimes several foci were present from each of which seizures could originate, the electrical signs alternating between one hemisphere and the other. Such seizures were always symptomatic of a cerebral lesion, most commonly birth damage and it was suggested (on analogy with the results of experiments in kittens) that the seizures depended on the activity of the hippocampus, which was the only effective structure sufficiently well organized at birth. Several types of generalized seizure were possible at later stages of childhood, including the petit mal absence, commonly with the "3 per second spike-wave" (see below), a type of "tonic" seizure (corresponding to a "grand mal" attack without the clonic phenomena) and a variety of other seizures, including the "petit mal variant" of Gibbs, which Passouant and Cadilhac thought should not be considered definite clinical entities as the EEG was so variable, ranging from a well-organized "absence" form at one extreme through slow and irregular spike-wave complexes to mixed slow waves and spikes (hypsarrhythmia) at the other. That the "infantile spasms" usually associated with the latter pattern should also not be considered a specific disease entity was suggested by Millichap et al. (1962) since almost any of the known causes of epilepsy in childhood could be held responsible. EEG, clinical and other aspects of infantile spasms are comprehensively dealt with in an excellent monograph by Jeavons and Bower (1964). Various types of generalized tonic seizures in children were also discussed by Gastaut et al. (1963). These differed from those of the "grand mal" type of epilepsy in being of short duration (usually 10–20 seconds) and uncomplicated by postictal exhaustion or coma. The EEG invariably showed bilaterally synchronous and symmetrical abnormalities and during the actual seizure there would be a rapid desynchronization (i.e. flattening of the record) with or without the development of bilaterally synchronous rhythmic activity at about 10 c/s which might ultimately develop into a slow or spike-wave pattern. The interest of these observations is that they demonstrate the existence of varieties of generalized epilepsy which differ clinically and electrically from "grand mal" and "petit mal" and at the same time have sufficient points of resemblance to suggest that there may be some truth in the hypothesis (Gibbs and Gibbs, 1952, and see also Wilder and Schmidt, 1965) that the spike-wave pattern reflects a more or less successful inhibition or restraint of the development of a truly generalized convulsive seizure. Three features at least influence the outcome of the initial process capable of progressing into a generalized seizure, the degree of development of the brain, the pathology and the inhibitory propensity. The relative importance of these in any given type of seizure and in any particular EEG pattern is at present almost impossible to elucidate and much more extensive investigation is needed, including the long-term follow-up with ultimate neuropathological studies such as that of Margerison and Corsellis (1966).

Gastaut et al. (1962b) describe two varieties of "hemiconvulsive seizures" which do not reflect a strictly unilateral epilepsy since both, the "hemi-grand mal" and the "hemiclonic" seizure can involve one side of the body or the other and the phenomena of a single seizure in the latter may alternate between the two sides. The EEG in these varieties is, broadly speaking, a unilateral version of what would be expected in a bilateral attack of the same variety, that is continuous (in the tonic phase) and interrupted (in the clonic phase) activity at about 10/sec in the "hemi-grand mal" seizure, and some variety of slow or spike-slow complexes in the "hemiclonic" seizure. These seizures may occur in children who have definite evidence of a cerebral lesion (and in particular those who showed in early life what Gastaut calls the HH syndrome—hemiconvulsions with hemiplegia—the final outcome when epileptic seizures appear to be permanently established being called the HHE syndrome), and they may also occur in the absence of any neurological or radiological signs of a diffuse or localized lesion. As Gastaut points out, it is important to recognize that not all "unilateral" seizures are "Jacksonian" and more than a unilateral seizure pattern is needed before a surgical operation is seriously to be considered.

Temporal lobe epilepsy is commonly thought of as a late adolescent and adult phenomenon, but Chao et al. (1962) stated that it was found in 15 per cent of epileptic patients under 15 seen at their clinic. They used purely clinical features for the diagnosis (e.g. aura

of gastric discomfort or fear, presence of various autonomic phenomena, a history of complex automatisms etc.) and found that about
60 per cent of these children had EEG abnormalities in the temporal
region. However, no adequate details of the EEG findings are given
and, since another 94 patients said not to have temporal lobe seizures
had such EEG abnormalities, the exact significance of the report
is not at all clear. There is no doubt that far too little is known about
the early history of those patients who ultimately, in late youth or
early adult life, are diagnosed as having temporal lobe epilepsy, but
such knowledge will only come when extensive clinical, electroencephalographic etc., examinations are made on many more children
than can be done at present, and when a more thorough follow-up
is also practised.

THE SPIKE-WAVE PHENOMENON

The recent discussion by Williams (1965) on the part played by
the upper brain stem in generalized epilepsy stimulates interest in
the spike-wave phenomenon as it appears likely that the association,
in petit mal, of loss of consciousness and the bilaterally synchronous
spike-wave pattern is an important factor in development of the
concept of centrencephalic epilepsy (Penfield and Jasper, 1954).
Jasper and Droogleever-Fortuyn (1947) and Hunter and Jasper
(1949) showed that both the "absence" and the bilateral spike-wave
bursts could be induced to appear in animals by electrical stimulation
of the mesial parts of the thalamus but reports from other laboratories (e.g. Ingvar, 1955) cast some doubt on the diencephalic
origin of such seizures. Few observations were made in human
beings, though Williams (1953) suggested that the spike component
was of thalamic origin whereas the slow wave was cortical. Weir
(1965) considered the phenomenon to be much more complex than
a simple two component pattern and suggested that the spike-wave
complex had certain resemblances to evoked cortical potentials.
This is likely as there appears to be no doubt that the potential
changes recorded as "spike-wave" in the scalp EEG actually arise
in the neurones of the cortex, though presumably as a result of
subcortical influence. The complex also differs in form in different
parts of the cortex.

The fact that spike-wave complexes are common in childhood
epilepsy but much rarer in adults led to a belief that the phenomenon
was essentially a property of the immature brain. This belief received
some support from the work of Guerrero-Figueroa et al. (1963)
which reported the effects of implantation of crystalline aluminium

oxide into various subcortical and cortical areas of kittens and adult cats. Only implantation into the intralaminar nuclei and reticular formation of kittens not more than 30 days old led to the development of 3/sec spikewave complexes and of a behavioural "absence."

However, Pollen et al. (1963) showed that the spike-wave pattern could be produced in more adult cats by stimulation of the intra-laminar system of the thalamus provided the animal was in a critical level of arousal, i.e. awake but slightly drowsy. This recalls the well-known observation in children with petit mal that spike-wave complexes readily appear when the patient is mentally relaxed but not when he is aroused, as by a sudden noise or painful stimulus. Pollen pointed out that in spite of these findings the initial discharge of petit mal epilepsy need not begin in the intralaminar system (which is relatively small in human beings) and reported a personal communication from Perot and Jasper to the effect that the midbrain was a more likely origin. This appears to have been confirmed by Weir (1964) who found in the cat that brief trains of stimuli at 3 per second applied to the mesencephalic reticular formation could lead to spike-wave production in the cortex and to an arrest reaction with head nodding, eyeball flutter and facial twitching. Both Pollen (loc. cit.) and Weir make the point that facial twitching and eye movements, both commonly seen in human petit mal attacks, do not follow from thalamic stimulation, which is another reason for believing that the midbrain plays a more fundamental part in human minor epilepsy than does the thalamus. Two other reports on the artificial production of the spike-wave pattern are of interest, though mainly in view of possible future developments. The first by Morillo and Baylor (1964) concerns the effects on cerebral electrical activity of intravenous injection of a quinazolone derivative, a procedure which may be of importance in micro-electrode studies. The second by Servít et al. (1965) is concerned with the frog brain, the relatively simple structure of which may more readily lend itself to studies of the pattern than does the mammalian brain.

Experimental work in human beings has been mainly concerned with assessing loss of various functions during bursts of the spike-wave phenomenon. Though both the patient and an observer may be aware of an actual lapse of consciousness (absence), neither may notice any very definite changes during a brief burst of spike-wave. However, in appropriate circumstances loss of function can be observed in relation to such short bursts though the time relations of the functional and EEG phenomena are not necessarily the same.

For example, Goldie and Green (1961) showed that a patient could continue speaking during the first 3 seconds of a spike-wave burst and perceive speech a second or so before the burst ended, though he might not be able to resume speech for some seconds after the end of the burst. Tizard and Margerison (1963a and b) showed that the most sensitive correlate of the spike-wave phenomenon was response time, slowing being found during bursts lasting only half a second. With longer bursts errors of omission also occurred. Davidoff and Johnson (1964) also found that the longer bursts were more likely to be associated with functional deficits. More complicated experiments were reported by Mirsky and van Buren (1965), the results of whose continuance performance test suggested that reception of information, motor output and an integrative process all suffered during spike wave bursts. These authors also confirmed a finding by Jus and Jus (1962) that a retrograde amnesia occurred in association with the burst, and that of Goldie and Green (*loc. cit.*) in relation to the tendency for dissociation of behavioural and electrographic phenomena.

These results indicate that the spike-wave burst should always be regarded as a truly ictal and not as an inter-ictal phenomenon analogous to a cortical spike focus. Also, the dissociation of effects in relation to the burst is perhaps evidence of incompletely related subcortical and cortical seizure activity and thus might be considered as confirmatory of a "deep" origin to the seizure.

Though deep midline lesions are far less likely to be associated with epilepsy than are lesions of the cerebral hemispheres (Williams, 1965), some reports of coincidence of such lesions and spike-wave complexes have recently appeared. For example Ajmone-Marsan and Lewis (1960) reviewed 13 cases and concluded that their findings supported a primary brain-stem role in the production of the EEG pattern. Scherman and Abraham (1963) drew a similar conclusion from four cases of precocious puberty with spike-wave in the EEG.

Taken all together there is thus a considerable body of evidence that would place the original disturbance responsible for the petit mal seizure deep within the brain, and probably in the brain stem. However, almost all this evidence depends on the assumption that the spike-wave of experimental epilepsy is closely related to, if not identical with, the spike-wave of human epilepsy. As Starzl *et al.* (1953) showed, spike-wave can in some circumstances be a purely cortical event and one must conclude that the final demonstration of the origin of the "petit mal discharge" is still wanting.

14 AND 6 PER SECOND POSITIVE SPIKES

Gibbs and Gibbs (1951, 1952) reported a relationship between EEG phenomena, which they called "14 and 6 per second positive spikes" and a clinical syndrome to which they gave the name "thalamic and hypothalamic epilepsy." The positive spikes are most frequently seen in adolescents and young adults, they occur in short bursts, are most prominent in the temporo-parietal areas and are readily disclosed by unipolar recording during light sleep. The epilepsy "is not what most neurologists and pediatricians call epilepsy" (Gibbs and Gibbs, 1963a) but is "a specific form of epilepsy, arising from a part of the brain which is not extremely convulsive but which . . . produces a less specific, generally milder and less incapacitating symptomatology than the previously recognized classical forms of epilepsy" (Gibbs and Gibbs, 1963b). The symptomatology includes episodic sensory, visceral, vegetative and emotional (behavioural) phenomena.

The existence of the "14 and 6" phenomenon as an electrographic entity is now widely accepted (see Henry, 1963 for a comprehensive review of published data), but its physiological basis is obscure.

Numerous reports have appeared concerning correlation of 14 and 6 per second positive spikes and clinical states, but even so Henry (1963) had to conclude that the real clinical significance of the pattern was anything but clear. Recent publications show evidence of attempts at more critical experimental methods than has been common in the past, but no very definite conclusions can be drawn. Friedlander (1964) found no 14 and 6 per second positive spikes at all in the EEGs of a group of young prisoners, each of whom had the symptoms said to be commonly associated with this pattern. However, a large number of his subjects were having treatment with anticonvulsant drugs and, since it is claimed by Gibbs and Gibbs (1963a) that anticonvulsants are highly effective in the treatment of thalamic and hypothalamic epilepsy, the results may be invalid. Small and Small (1964) compared 25 patients with 14 and 6 per second positive spikes in the EEG and 25 patients without such spikes (all 50 being referrals to the EEG laboratory of an acute intensive psychiatric hospital) and were unable to confirm that this EEG phenomenon had any significance. Hughes et al. (1965) carried out EEG examinations on 135 patients, all of whom had been referred by a psychiatrist as cases of behaviour disorder and "possible candidates for the positive spike phenomenon". Of these,

50 did in fact have positive spikes, 50 had normal records and the remaining 35 had abnormalities other than positive spikes. The only very significant differences between those with positive spikes and those with normal EEGs were that the former had attacks of more sudden onset, that they were more remorseful after the act and that they were more blunted emotionally.

Walter and Grossman (1963) described the 14 and 6 per second positive spike phenomenon as "a signal in a search for significance" and so it remains. Until much more definite evidence is available than at the present time it should be regarded as a feature to be expected under certain conditions in the EEG of the healthy and unhealthy alike, but one which, neither in its presence nor its absence has any very definite clinical significance.

PROGNOSIS

The prognostic value of the EEG in epilepsy can be discussed in several ways, e.g. in relation to the possibility of the development of epilepsy after a head injury or cerebral infection etc., in relation to the possible outcome in a patient who already has epileptic seizures and in relation to the effects of a surgical operation for the relief of epilepsy. The last has been mentioned above in the discussion of electrocorticography.

Post-traumatic epilepsy was thoroughly discussed by Marshall and Walker (1961) who also reported their findings in a large number of men with head injuries dating from the second World War. 80 of these had EEGs taken within 6 months of injury and again 5 years later, and no significant differences emerged whether epilepsy ultimately occurred or not. 195 had EEGs taken 5–9 years after the injury, and when these were grouped according to whether the subjects had epilepsy or not no essential differences between the groups could be seen. Marshall and Walker concluded that there was no satisfactory evidence that the EEG will indicate the possibility of, the presence of, or the absence of a post-traumatic epilepsy. In a later publication, Walker (1962) suggested that the only valid conclusion one could make was that a normal record after a head injury indicated little brain damage and hence a slight chance of the development of epilepsy. Masquin and Courjon (1963) found that a return to normal of the EEG in the early post-traumatic period was not necessarily a favourable sign, indicating that it is probably unwise to place much prognostic reliance on a normal EEG if it is taken more than a few hours after the injury. They also made the point that the most complex prognostic problem was that of the patient who had already developed epileptic seizures but who had a normal EEG.

According to Gibbs *et al.* (1963) it is quite the opposite with cerebral palsy in children. They discussed the EEGs of 324 patients most of whom were seen for the first time at the age of 3 or earlier, at which time none had had seizures, and about 3 times later at approximately 2 year intervals. The main findings were that after the age of 2 a normal EEG almost invariably meant that epilepsy would not develop, and that those who did in fact have spikes in the EEG before 2 were more likely to have epileptic seizures than those whose spikes developed at a later age. Pedersen (1964) followed 80 cases of primary aseptic encephalitis (children and adults) for about 5 years from the acute or subacute stage and found a higher incidence of EEG abnormalities in those who developed epilepsy. He found that the initial EEG pattern was of no prognostic value, but an increasing abnormality was seen only in those patients who ultimately had epileptic seizures.

Lundervold (1964) examined 78 epileptic children on admission to hospital and again 5–15 years later. Of 22 patients who had normal EEGs on first admission 18 ultimately became seizure free and of 11 with a severely abnormal EEG on first admission 8 became seizure free. However, the findings reported in an earlier publication (Lundervold and Jabbour, 1962) indicated that a normal first (e.g. pretreatment) EEG was much more likely to be found in an ultimately seizure-free group than in an unimproved group, and vice versa with a severely abnormal first EEG. Hertoft (1963) followed 50 patients with petit mal epilepsy for an average of almost 13 years after the first attack. He found that of the 24 who became seizure-free 20 per cent had normal EEG records, 50 per cent continuing to have definite spike-wave bursts.

It is apparent that little prognostic reliance can be placed on a single EEG record in these cases, and comparison of such a record taken at an early admission with one taken a number of years later is only likely to be fruitful if many factors are taken into consideration other than those generally included in an "improved" or "unimproved" assessment. Prognosis in epileptic patients is likely to remain hazardous until very much more is known about the actual meaning of "abnormalities" in the inter-ictal record than at present. It is similar with the problem of epilepsy arising as a result of some cerebral lesion (with a possible exception in very young children): too little is known about the basis of electrical abnormalities to separate (if this is possible) those which reflect an abnormality of function which can also manifest itself in some epileptic phenomenon from those which are associated with other types of cerebral dysfunction—e.g. paresis, dyskinesia and dementia.

References

AJMONE-MARSAN, C. (1963). *Electroenceph. clin. Neurophysiol.*, **15**, 197.

AJMONE-MARSAN, C., and ABRAHAM, K. (1960). "A Seizure Atlas". *Electroenceph. clin. Neurophysiol.*, **12**, Suppl. 15.

AJMONE-MARSAN, C., and LEWIS, W. R. (1960). *Neurology*, **10**, 922.

AJMONE-MARSAN, C., and RALSTON, B. L. (1957). *The Epileptic Seizure*. Springfield, Ill., Thomas.

BATES, J. A. V. (1961). *Excerpta med., int. congr. series*, **37**, 62.

BENNET, D. R. (1963). *Neurology*, **13**, 953.

BICKFORD, R. G. (1949). *Electroenceph. clin. Neurophysiol.*, **1**, 126.

BICKFORD, R. G., SEM-JACOBSEN, C. W., WHITE, P. T., and DALY, D. (1952). *Electroenceph. clin. Neurophysiol.*, **4**, 275.

BLADIN, P. F. (1963). *Epilepsia*, **4**, 151.

CHAO, D., SEXTON, J. A., and PARDO L. S. S. (1962)., *J. Pediat.*, **60**, 686.

CHATRIAN, G. E., and PEREZ-BORJA, C. (1964). *Electroenceph. clin. Neurophysiol.*, **17**, 71.

CHATRIAN, G. E., and PETERSEN, M. C. (1960). *Electroenceph. clin. Neurophysiol.*, **12**, 715.

CHATRIAN, G. E., DODGE, H. W., PETERSEN, M. C., and BICKFORD, R. G. (1959a). *Electroenceph. clin. Neurophysiol.*, **11**, 165.

CHATRIAN, G. E., POLLACK, C. S., and PETERSEN, M. C. (1959b). *Electroenceph. clin. Neurophysiol.*, **11**, 358.

COCEANI, F., LIBMAN, I., and GLOOR, P. (1966). *Electroenceph. clin. Neurophysiol.*, **20**, 542.

CRANDALL, P. H., WALTER, R. D., and RAND, R. W. (1963). *J. Neurosurg.*, **20**, 827.

CURE, C., RASMUSSEN, T., and JASPER, H. (1948). *Arch. neurol. psychiat.*, **59**, 691.

DAVIDOFF, R. A., and JOHNSON, L. C. (1964). *Electroenceph. clin. Neurophysiol.*, **16**, 343.

DAVISON, K. (1965). *Electroenceph. clin. Neurophysiol.*, **19**, 298.

DELGADO, J. M. R. (1952). *Yale J. Biol. Med.*, **24**, 351.

DRIVER, M. V. (1962). *Electroenceph. clin. Neurophysiol.*, **14**, 359.

DRIVER, M. V., FALCONER, M. A., and SERAFETINIDES, E. A. (1964). *Neurology*, **14**, 455.

ECHLIN, F. A., and BATTISTA, A. (1963). *Arch. neurol.*, **9**, 154.

FALCONER, M. A., DRIVER, M. V., and SERAFETINIDES, E. A. (1962). *Brain*, **85**, 521.

FISCHER-WILLIAMS, M., and COOPER, R. A. (1963). *Electroenceph. clin. Neurophysiol.*, **15**, 568.

FRIEDLANDER, W. J. (1964). *Dis. nerv. Syst.*, **25**, 370.

GASTAUT, H. (1950). *Electroenceph. clin. Neurophysiol.*, **2**, 249.

GASTAUT, H. (1964). *Epilepsia*, **5**, 297.

GASTAUT, H., and FISCHER-WILLIAMS, M. (1959). In *Handbook of Physiology* ed. Field, J., Section I, Vol. 1, Baltimore, Williams & Wilkins.

GASTAUT, H., and GIBSON, W. C. (1960). *Aerospace Med.*, **31**, 531.

GASTAUT, H., REGIS, H., and BOSTEM, F. (1962a). *Epilepsia*, **3**, 438.
GASTAUT, H., ROGER, J., and FAIDHERBE, J. (1962b). *Epilepsia*, **3**, 56.
GASTAUT, H., ROGER, J., and OUAHCHI, S. (1963). *Epilepsia*, **4**, 15.
GASTAUT, H., VIGOUROUX, M., and TREVISAN, C. (1957). *Rev. neurol.*, **97**, 37.
GIBBS, E. L., and GIBBS, F. A. (1951). *Neurology*, **1**, 136.
GIBBS, F. A., and GIBBS, E. L. (1952). *Atlas of Electroencephalography*, Vol. II, Cambridge, Mass. Addison-Wesley Press.
GIBBS, F. A., and GIBBS, E. L. (1963a). *J. Neuropsychiat.*, **4**, 287.
GIBBS, F. A., and GIBBS, E. L. (1963b). *Electroenceph. clin. Neurophysiol.*, **15**, 553.
GIBBS, F. A., GIBBS, E. L., and FUSTER, B. (1947). *Trans. Amer. neurol. Ass.*, **72**, 180.
GIBBS, F. A., GIBBS, E. L., PERLSTEIN, M. A., and RICH, C. L. (1963). *Neurology*, **13**, 143.
GLOOR, P., RASMUSSEN, T., GARRETSON, H., and MAROUN, F. (1964). *Electroenceph. clin. Neurophysiol.*, **17**, 322.
GOLDENSOHN, E. S. (1962). *Bull. N.Y. Acad. Med.*, **38**, 653.
GOLDIE, L., and GREEN, J. M. (1959). *Brain*, **82**, 505.
GOLDIE, L., and GREEN, J. M. (1961). *Nature*, **191**, 200.
GOTOH, F., MEYER, J. S., and TAKAGI, Y. (1965). *Arch. neurol.*, **12**, 410.
GREEN, J. B. (1963). *Neurology*, **13**, 192.
GREEN, J. R., and SCHEETZ, D. G. (1964). *Arch. neurol.*, **10**, 135.
GUERRERO-FIGUEROA, R., BARROS, A., VERSTER, F., and HEATH, R. G. (1963). *Arch. Neurol.*, **9**, 297.
GUERRERO-FIGUEROA, R., BARROS, A., HEATH, R. G., and GONZALEZ, G. (1964). *Epilepsia*, **5**, 112.
HENRY, C. E. (1963). In Glaser, G. H. (Ed.). *EEG and Behaviour*. London, Basic Books.
HERTOFT, P. (1963). *Epilepsia*, **4**, 298.
HILL, J. D. N., and PARR, G. (1963). *Electroencephalography*, London, Macdonald.
HUGHES, J. R., MEANS, E. D., and STELL, B. S. (1965). *Electroenceph. clin. Neurophysiol.*, **18**, 349.
HUNTER, J., and JASPER, H. H. (1949). *Electroenceph. clin. Neurophysiol.*, **1**, 305.
INGVAR, D. H. (1955). *Acta physiol. Scand.*, **33**, 137.
JASPER, H. H., and DROOGLEEVER-FORTUYN, J. (1947). *Res. Publ. Ass. nerv. ment. Dis.*, **26**, 272.
JASPER, H. H., ARFEL-CAPDEVILLE, G., and RASMUSSEN, T. (1961). *Epilepsia*, **2**, 130.
JEAVONS, P. M., and BOWER, B. D. (1964). *Infantile Spasms*, London, Heinemann.
JUS, A., and JUS, K. (1962). *Arch. gen. Psychiat.*, **6**, 163.
KENNEDY, W. A. (1959). *Brain*, **82**, 147.
KENNEDY, W. A., and DRIVER, M. V. (1962). *Electroenceph. clin. Neurophysiol.*, **14**, 790.
KENNEDY, W. A., and HILL, D. (1958). *J. Neurol. Neurosurg. Psychiat.*, **21**, 24.
KENNEDY, W. A., and MARLEY, E. (1959). *Electroenceph. clin. Neurophysiol.*, **11**, 59.
KILOH, L. G., and OSSELTON, J. W. (1966). *Clinical electroencephalography*, 2nd ed. London, Butterworths.
KOOI, K. A., GÜVENER, A. M., TUPPER, C. J., and BAGCHI, B. K. (1964). *Neurology*, **14**, 1029.

LISHMAN, W. A., SYMONDS, C. P., WHITTY, C. W. M., and WILLISON, R. G. (1962), *Brain*, **85**, 93.

LISKE, E. A., and FORSTER, F. M. (1964). *Neurology*, **14**, 41.

LISKE, E. A., GILSON, W. E., and FORSTER, F. M. (1962). *J. Amer. med. Ass.*, **182**, 582.

LLEWELLYN, R. C., and HEATH, R. G. (1962). *Confinia neurol.*, **22**, 223.

LUNDERVOLD, A. (1964). *Epilepsia*, **5**, 33.

LUNDERVOLD, A., and JABBOUR, J. T. (1962). *J. Pediat.*, **60**, 220.

LYBERI, G., and LAST, S. L. (1956). *Electroenceph. clin. Neurophysiol.*, **8**, 711.

MAGNUS, O., DE VET, A. C., VAN DER MAREL, A., and MEYER, E. (1962). *Devel. med. and child Neurol.*, **4**, 35.

MARGERISON, J. H., and CORSELLIS, J. A. N. (1966). *Brain*, **89**, 499.

MARSHALL, C., and WALKER, A. E. (1961). *Epilepsia*, **2**, 138.

MASQUIN, A., and COURJON, J. (1963). *Epilepsia*, **4**, 285.

MAWDSLEY, C. (1961). *Lancet*, **1**, 190.

MAYO SYMPOSIUM (1953). *Proc. Mayo Clin.*, **145**.

MEDUNA, L. VON (1935). *Psych. neurol. Wochenschr.*, **37**, 317.

MERLIS, J. K., HENRIKSEN, G. F., and GROSSMAN, C. (1950). *Electroenceph. clin. Neurophysiol.*, **2**, 17.

MEWBURN, R. H., and GIBSON, W. C. (1963). *Canad. med. assoc. J.*, **88**, 641.

MEYER, J. S., and GOTOH, F. (1960). *Arch. neurol.*, **3**, 539.

MILLICHAP, J. G, BICKFORD, R. G., KLASS, D. W., and BACKUS, R. E. (1962). *Epilepsia*, **3**, 188.

MIRSKY, A. F., and VAN BUREN, J. M. (1965). *Electroenceph. clin. Neurophysiol.*, **18**, 334.

MORRELL, F. (1959). *Arch. Neurol.*, **1**, 141.

MORREL, F. (1960). *Epilepsia*, **1**, 538.

MORILLO, A., and BAYLOR, D. (1964). *Electroenceph. clin. Neurophysiol.*, **16**, 519.

NIEDERMEYER, E. (1965). *Arch. neurol.*, **12**, 625.

PALLIS, C., and LOUIS, S. (1961). *Lancet*, **1**, 188.

PAMPIGLIONE, G., and KERRIDGE, J. (1956). *J. Neurol., Neurosurg. Psychiat.*, **19**, 117.

PANTELAKIS, S. N., BOWER, B. D., and JONES, H. D. (1962). *Brit. med. J.*, **5,305** 633.

PASSOUANT, P., and CADILHAC, J. (1962). *Epilepsia*, **3**, 14.

PEDERSEN, E. (1964). *Epilepsia*, **5**, 43.

PENFIELD, W., and JASPER, H. (1954). *Epilepsy and the Functional Anatomy of the Human Brain*. London, Churchill.

PEREZ-BORJA, C., and RIVERS, M. H. (1963). *Electroenceph. clin. Neurophysiol.*, **15**, 588.

POLLEN, D. A., PEROT, P., and REID, K. H. (1963). *Electroenceph. clin. Neurophysiol.*, **15**, 1017.

POSKANZER, D. C., BROWN, A. E., and MILLER, H. (1962). *Brain*, **85**, 77.

PUTNAM, T. J., and MERRITT, H. H. (1937). *Science*, **85**, 525.

RALSTON, B. L. (1958). *Electroenceph. clin. Neurophysiol.*, **10**, 217.

RALSTON, B. L., and PAPATHEODOROU, C. A. (1960). *Electroenceph. clin. Neurophysiol.*, **12**, 297.

RODIN, E. A. (1964). *Epilepsia*, **5**, 21.

RODIN, E. A., LIU, Y., GONZALEZ, S., and DENNERLL, R. D. (1964). *IEEE Trans. Biomed. Eng.*, **11**, 19.

ROGINA, V., and SERAFETINIDES, E. A. (1962). *Electroenceph. clin. Neurophysiol.*, **14**, 376.

ROVIT, R. L., GLOOR, P., and RASMUSSEN, T. (1961a). *J. Neurosurg.*, **18**, 151.

ROVIT, R. L., GLOOR, P., and RASMUSSEN, T. (1961b). *Arch. neurol.*, **5**, 606.

SALZMAN, H. A., HEYMAN, A., and SIEKER, H. O. (1963). *New Eng. J. Med.*, **268**, 1431.

SCHERMAN, R. G., and ABRAHAM, K. (1963). *Electroenceph. clin. Neurophysiol.*, **15**, 559.

SELLDEN, U. (1964). *Acta neurol. Scand.* Suppl. 12, Vol. 40.

SERAFETINIDES, E. A., HOARE, R. D., and DRIVER, M. V. (1965a). *Brain*, **88**, 107.

SERAFETINIDES, E. A., DRIVER, M. V., and HOARE, R. D. (1965b). *Electroenceph. clin. Neurophysiol.*, **18**, 170.

SERVÍT, Z., MACHEK, J., and FISCHER, J. (1965). *Electroenceph. clin. Neurophysiol.*, **19**, 162.

SHERWOOD, S. L. (1962). *Arch. neurol.*, **6**, 49.

SILFVENIUS, H., GLOOR, P., and RASMUSSEN, T. (1964). *Epilepsia*, **5**, 307.

SMALL, J. G., and SMALL, I. F. (1964). *Arch. gen. psychiat.*, **11**, 645.

SMALL, J. G., STEVENS, J. R., and MILSTEIN, V. (1964). *J. nerv. ment. Dis.*, **138**, 146.

STARZL, T. E., NIEMER, W. T., DELL, M., and FORGRAVE, P. R. (1953). *J. Neuropath. exp. Neurol.*, **12**, 262.

STEVENS, J. R. (1962). *Arch. neurol.*, **7**, 330.

SYMPOSIUM ON INDOKLON (1962). *J. Neuropsychiat.*, **4**, 149.

TENGESDAL, M. (1963). *Acta neurol. Scand.*, **39**, Suppl. 4, 329.

TIZARD, B., and MARGERISON, J. H. (1963a). *Brit. J. soc. clin. psychol.*, **3**, 6.

TIZARD, B., and MARGERISON, J. H. (1963b). *J. Neurol. Neurosurg. Psychiat.*, **26**, 308.

TÜKEL, L., and JASPER, H. H. (1952). *Electroenceph. clin. Neurophysiol.*, **4**, 481.

ULETT, G. A., BROCKMAN, J. C., GLESER, G., and JOHNSON, A. (1955). *Electroenceph. clin. Neurophysiol.*, **7**, 597.

WADA, J. (1949). *Med. Biol. Tokyo*, **14**, 221.

WADA, J., and RASMUSSEN, T. (1960). *J. Neurosurg.*, **17**, 266.

WALKER, A. E. (1962). *World neurol.*, **3**, 185.

WALTER, R. D., and GROSSMAN, H. J. (1963). *Electroenceph. clin. Neurophysiol.*, **15**, 161.

WEIR, B. (1964). *Arch. neurol.*, **11**, 209.

WEIR, B. (1965). *Electroenceph. clin. Neurophysiol.*, **19**, 284.

WILDER, B. J., and SCHMIDT, R. P. (1965). *Epilepsia*, **6**, 297.

WILLIAMS, D. (1953). *Electroenceph. clin. Neurophysiol.*, **5**, 325.

WILLIAMS, D. (1965). *Brain*, **88**, 539.

ZISKIND, E., SJAARDEMA, H., and BERCEL, N. A. (1946). *Science*, **104**, 462.

CHAPTER 10

RECENT ADVANCES IN NEURORADIOLOGY

DAVID SUTTON

RECENT advances in the field of neuroradiology will be considered under the following headings:

1. Angiography.
2. Pneumography.
3. The Spine.
4. Ultrasonic Encephalography.
5. Isotope Encephalography.

ANGIOGRAPHY

The Deep Veins

In recent years increasing attention has been paid to the deep venous system of drainage of the brain and its displacement by expanding lesions. The normal radiological anatomy has been well known for many years and is illustrated in Fig. 23. The internal cerebral vein lies just lateral to the midline in the velum interpositum in the roof of the third ventricle. It is formed by the confluence of the vein of the septum pellucidum and of the strio-thalamic vein. This lies just behind the foramen of Monro. This point is usually referred to as the "venous angle". Other tributary veins also drain into the internal cerebral vein as shown in the diagram. The tributary veins commence at the margins of the ventricle where they receive the blood from the subependymal veins draining the cerebral white matter. Posteriorly the two internal cerebral veins unite just above and behind the pineal to form the great vein of Galen. This, together with the inferior sagittal sinus drains into the straight sinus. All these anatomical features are recognizable in a late phlebogram exposed towards the end of an angiographic series. The basal vein of Rosenthal is rather more variable but is also usually recognizable.

The internal cerebral vein and its main tributaries have a constant position in both lateral and antero-posterior projections. The displacement of these vessels is an important angiographic sign of the presence of a tumour. It is even more important that such angiographic evidence may be present though the arteries seem normal in

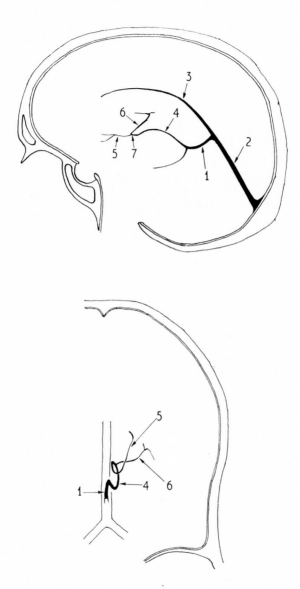

Figure 23*a and b.* (1) Vein of Galen. (2) Straight sinus. (3) Inferior sagittal sinus. (4) Internal cerebral vein. (5) Septal vein. (6) Strio-thalamic vein. (7) Venous angle.

position. This can happen with deep seated basal tumours, or with deep temporal lesions (Fig. 24). Thus careful examination of the disposition of the deep veins is now an essential part of a cerebral angiographic study.

The fact that the subependymal veins supplying the internal cerebral vein arise in the margins of the lateral ventricle enables us to assess the size of the ventricles at angiography (Fig. 25). Thus with a gross hydrocephalous the appearances are usually diagnostic. Local distortions of the ventricles can also be recognized from displacement of subependymal veins (Wolf and Huang, 1964).

Knowledge of the normal anatomy of the deep veins also permits a better assessment of the extent of large vascular tumours such as malignant gliomas, or of angiomatous malformations. Wolf and Huang (1964) have shown that abnormal veins of the white matter draining into the subependymal veins can be readily recognized at angiography.

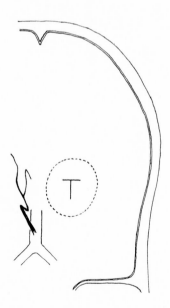

Figure 24. Displacement of the deep veins across the mid line with a thalamic tumour.

Cerebrovascular Insufficiency

There has been a considerable amount of angiographic work done in recent years on the problem involved in cerebral ischæmia and cerebrovascular insufficiency. Since Hutchinson and Yates (1957) first drew attention to atheromatous lesions of the vertebral arteries it has been generally recognized that atheromatous stenosis and thrombosis of the extracranial vessels is common and that multiple vessels may be involved. We have been particularly interested in this problem and our own findings confirm the general trend of other work in this field (Sutton and Davies, 1966).

We have examined over 300 cases of carotid insufficiency by simple carotid angiography. About two-thirds of these patients have had bilateral angiograms performed and in the patients where this has been done about 40 per cent were found to have bilateral lesions. The classical symptomatology of carotid insufficiency has been well described in the literature and has given rise to the mixed metaphors of "stuttering hemiplegia" or "cerebral claudication". It is important to realize, however, that a significant proportion of patients may present with misleading symptoms or may have no symptoms at all. We have seen many cases where the diagnosis of carotid thrombosis and even of bilateral carotid thrombosis came as a surprise to the referring neurologist.

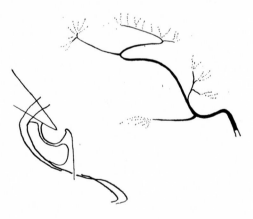

Figure 25. Subependymal veins (dotted) draining from the white matter and joining the deep veins at the margins of the ventricles. Their appearance enables the size and shape of the ventricle to be assessed from the angiogram.

In 1946 it was shown by Kubik and Adams that basilar thrombosis was not necessarily fatal and later the concept of "vertebrobasilar insufficiency" gained currency (Williams and Wilson, 1962). Unfortunately, the symptoms ascribed to such vertebrobasilar insufficiency are rather protean and numerous. The symptom occurring with most frequency is "attacks of giddiness". This was present in over 50 per cent of the cases described by Williams and Wilson.

The pathological and clinical evidence have led workers in this field to suggest that the radiological demonstration of all the extracranial vessels is desirable when cerebrovascular insufficiency is suspected. We have now performed over 600 arch aortograms in cases of "cerebrovascular insufficiency" and have confirmed *in vivo* the pathological evidence suggesting that multiple lesions are common.

Techniques of Examination

Four-vessel angiography is necessary to outline the extracranial vessels. The different methods available have been:

Venous Angiocardiography. For this method a large bolus of contrast is injected into the venous system. After circulation through the right side of the heart and the pulmonary circulation the bolus reaches the left side of the heart and the systemic circulation. Films are exposed as the contrast passes through the aortic arch and great vessels. This method has the defect of providing rather weak opacification of the major vessels unless excessive doses of contrast are used. It has largely been replaced by direct injection into the aortic arch.

Retrograde Brachial Arteriography. Brachial arteriography with forced retrograde injection of contrast into the right brachial artery after percutaneous puncture of the artery has been widely used in the United States, but has found little acceptance in Europe. This method will permit visualization of the right carotid and right vertebral arteries, but further arterial punctures are usually necessary to show the left vertebral and left common carotid arteries well.

Arch Aortography. This is performed by percutaneous catheterization of the aorta either from the femoral artery, or from the right axillary artery. In either case the catheter tip is manipulated to enter the ascending aorta. We prefer the trans-femoral approach though the trans-axillary approach is used as an alternative, particularly in patients with severe atheroma of the iliacs. 40 ml of concentrated contrast medium (Triosil 75 per cent or Conray 480) is injected into the ascending aorta within two seconds. Rapid serial films are obtained of the aortic arch and great vessels, the exposures being made within 3–4 seconds.

This method usually provides excellent visualization of the great vessels arising from the aortic arch, of the whole of the cervical vertebral arteries, and of the carotids as far as the base of the skull, including their bifurcations (Fig. 26).

In skilled hands the procedure can be carried out with little upset to the patient and we normally perform it under local anæsthesia and basal premedication only. In poor-risk patients, however, and many of these patients have generalized arterial disease, the investigation should be ordered with caution. We have had one death in

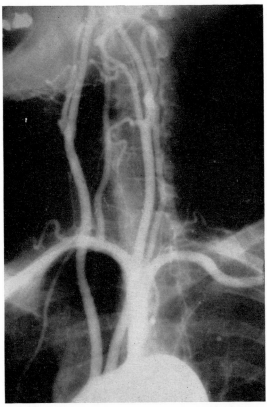

Figure 26. Arch aortogram by right transaxillary catheterisation. There is an anomalous right subclavian artery arising distally on the arch. The vertebrals and carotids are normal.

TABLE 6. RELATIONSHIP BETWEEN THE CLINICAL SYNDROMES AND THE SITE OF THE RADIOLOGICAL LESIONS

CLINICAL SYNDROME	SITE OF RADIOLOGICAL LESIONS (percentages)						CASES TOTAL No.
	Carotid	Vertebral	Both	Subclavian Steal	Atheroma	Nil	
Carotid insufficiency	42·1%	9·5%	6·0%	2·3%	18·0%	22·1%	88
Basilar insufficiency	16·01%	16·5%	6·0%	8·8%	23·0%	29·7%	187
Caroticobasilar insufficiency	17·3%	19·2%	25·0%	13·5%	7·7%	17·3%	54
Ischaemia of arm only							1*
Total all syndromes	23·0%	15·6%	9·0%	7·9%	18·8%	25·7%	330

* Denotes a case of subclavian steal who had ischaemia of his arm without cerebral symptoms.

our last 500 patients. This resulted from acute thrombosis of a severely stenosed carotid artery. The thrombosis occurred 6 hours after angiography and was presumably precipated by the hypotensive reaction due to the investigation. Thrombosis at the site of the catheter introduction is another danger. We have seen ischæmic legs three times in about two thousand transfemoral catheterizations. All our cases recovered, though surgery to remove local clot was necessary in one case.

Clinical Aspects

Figs. 27 and 28 illustrate the total number of thrombosis and stenoses found in a consecutive series of 330 cases examined by Sutton and Davies (1966) and clinically diagnosed as various forms of cerebrovascular insufficiency. The frequent discovery of multiple lesions and of lesions not apparently related to the clinical symptoms the patient complained of raises many problems (Table 6).

It is clear from this study that there is frequently a poor correlation between the anatomical obstructive lesions and the clinical state of the patient.

Surgeons have tended to take a simple view of the problems raised. They have argued, with some reason, that where a partial obstruction to a major cerebral blood vessel is shown, then restoration of normal flow by surgery is a reasonable procedure which must improve total cerebral blood flow. It has also been claimed that removal of an atheromatous stenosis is prophylactic in as much as it will prevent a later thrombosis which may produce a severe deficit.

On the other hand the natural history of extracranial vascular disease has been inadequately studied. There is good evidence from studies of pathology that stenoses and thromboses occur frequently in symptomless patients and there is now in vivo angiographic evidence that extensive disease can be present with little disability (Fig. 29).

There seems as yet no method of deciding which patient is going to produce severe symptoms when a vessel finally occludes. Thus in the present state of our knowledge the case for surgery in stenotic lesions of the extracranial vessels seems fairly sound.

The answer to some of the problems posed by the above observations seems to lie in the collateral circulation. Thus Alpers et al. (1964) have shown that congenital anomalies of the circle of Willis are extremely common. Absence or hypoplasia of one or more posterior communicating arteries is present in about one-third of

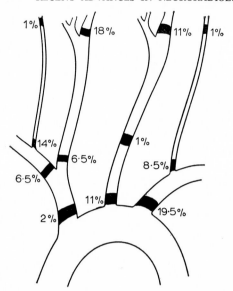

Figure 27. Site of 93 thromboses in a series of 330 cases.

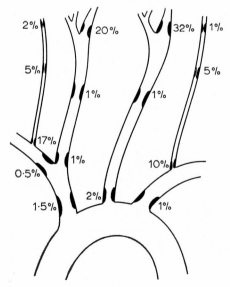

Figure 28. Site of 170 stenoses in a series of 330 cases.
(*Figs.* 27 *and* 28 *reproduced from Sutton and Davies* (1966).)

normal individuals. Anomalies of the anterior communicating arteries are less frequent but also occur. Since collateral circulation depends so much on the circle of Willis a defective circle is obviously of great importance and relevance where a patient suffers occlusion of the four major extra cranial vessels. On the other hand, an efficient circle of Willis will allow a good collateral circulation. Apart from the circle of Willis our angiographic studies have also shown numerous other collateral pathways.

These are illustrated in Fig. 30. The different collaterals vary in importance in individual cases, depending on the site of the obstructive

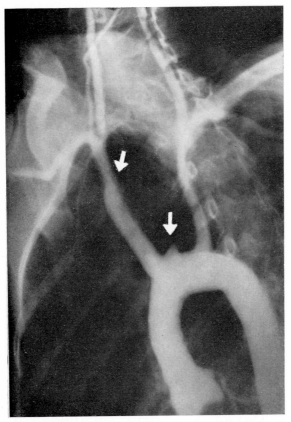

Figure 29. Arch aortogram showing complete thrombosis of right common carotid and left common carotid arteries.

(*Reproduced from Sutton and Davies* (1966))

lesion or lesions, their rapidity of onset, and the individual vascular anatomy. Hawkins (1966) has recently reviewed the cerebral collateral pathways, and it is clear that most people have a considerable potential for coping with both extracranial and intracranial vascular obstruction.

Apart from the circle of Willis the following alternative pathways are important and the flow in them may be in either direction.

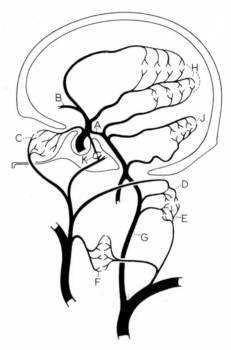

Figure 30. The collateral pathways in cerebro vascular insufficiency. (A and B)—Posterior communicating and anterior communicating arteries of the circle of Willis. (C)—Communications between maxillary and ophthalmic artery. (D)—Communication between muscular branches of the vertebral and the occipital artery. (E)—Communication between the vertebral and ascending cervical arteries. (F)—Communication between the inferior thyroid and superior thyroid arteries of the same and opposite sides. (G)—The vertebral artery providing retrograde flow to the subclavian (subclavian steal). (H)—Pial anastomoses between terminal branches of the anterior cerebral, middle cerebral, and posterior cerebral arteries. (J)—Pial anastomoses in the posterior fossa. (K)—Meningeal anastomoses and rete mirabile.

1. Between the maxillary branch of the external carotid and the ophthalmic branch of the internal carotid.

2. Between the occipital branch of the external carotid and the muscular branches of the vertebral.

3. Between the cervical branches of the subclavian and branches of the external carotid.

4. Between the cervical branches of the subclavian and the muscular branches of the vertebral.

5. Pial anastomosis between the anterior, middle, and posterior cerebral arteries and also between the major vessels in the posterior fossa.

6. Between the middle meningeal and the pial branches of the internal carotid.

7. "Rete mirabile", a remnant of the primitive communications at the base of the skull between the external and internal carotid systems.

8. Persistence of large communications between the internal carotid and the basilar ("trigeminal artery", or carotid basilar anastomosis etc.).

Subclavian Steal

This Americanism is the term which has gained general currency to describe the unusual situation where the proximal part of a subclavian artery is occluded and the ipsilateral vertebral artery provides a collateral to the arm (Fig. 31). Thus when the first part of the left subclavian artery is occluded the pressure in the left subclavian at the origin of the left vertebral artery falls to zero. The pressure at the distal end of the artery where it joins the normal right vertebral is systemic. There is then a pressure gradient from the top of the vertebral artery down to its origin, and blood refluxes to the left arm. It is postulated that this "shunt" diverts blood from the brain and thus produces cerebrovascular insufficiency.

We have now performed angiography on 30 patients of this type. As in most other reported series the majority of our cases have affected the left subclavian, but we have also seen some patients with a right subclavian steal, due either to occlusion of the innominate artery or of the right subclavian origin.

Some workers have claimed that exercising the affected arm might produce symptoms by increasing the amount of diverted blood but there is little *in vivo* evidence to support this contention. In most of our cases multiple extracranial lesions were present and in others the diagnosis was suggested not by the presence of cerebral

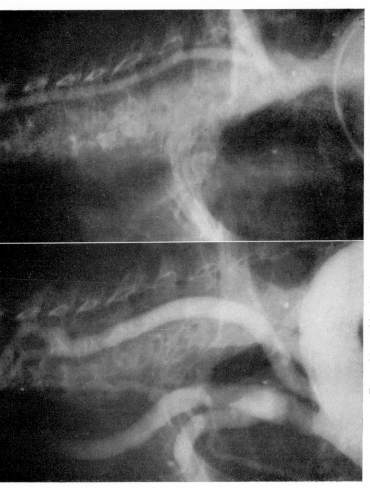

Figure 31a *and b.* Arch aortogram showing "subclavian steal".
(Reproduced from Sutton and Davies (1966).)

symptoms but by differences of pulse pressure in the two arms.

In our patients there has been a poor correlation between cerebral symptoms and the presence of a subclavian steal. Our evidence suggests that a "steal" may aggravate a poor cerebral flow due to other lesions but is rarely a cause of symptoms in itself. Indeed the finding of subclavian "steal" was a surprise in several of our patients in whom other lesions were suspected.

Subarachnoid Hæmorrhage

Recent studies have shown that a very high degree of accuracy in the diagnosis of the site and nature of the lesion in cases of sub-arachnoid hæmorrhage can be achieved by careful and systematic angiography. For many years most workers practised unilateral angiography if there were localizing signs, and bilateral carotid angiography if there were none. Where the findings were negative vertebral angiography might be proceeded with. Policy varies in different centres, and vertebral arteriography was frequently performed at a few centres, but only rarely at others.

After bilateral carotid angiography a lesion can be demonstrated in about 75 per cent of cases and the findings were very similar in the major series of Walsh (1956) and of Sutton and Trickey (1962).

In the 1018 cases listed above, aneurysms were shown in just over half the cases, angiomas in about 10 per cent, and hæmatomas in a similar percentage. The hæmatomas were presumed to arise from rupture of an atheromatous vessel, or of an aneurysm or angioma too small to visualize.

The 25 per cent incidence of negative findings can be appreciably reduced in cases where vertebral angiography is performed. Thus

TABLE 7. FINDINGS AFTER BILATERAL CAROTID ANGIOGRAPHY

	WALSH (461 cases) per cent	SUTTON AND TRICKEY GROUP 1 (557 cases) per cent
Aneurysms	54	54
Angiomas	11.5	7.5
Hæmatomas	7.5	12.5
Tumour	0	1
Negative	27	25

Spatz and Bull (1957) found lesions in 16 out of 44 cases, and Sutton and Trickey found lesions in 29 out of 77 patients after unilateral vertebral angiography (see Table 8).

Sutton and Trickey (1962) also showed that the incidence of positive diagnostic results could be improved by injecting the second vertebral artery after both carotids and one vertebral had been injected with negative results.

They injected the second vertebral artery in 25 of the 48 cases where unilateral vertebral angiography was negative and showed lesions in 7 patients. This is because, in a small proportion of cases, an aneurysm or other lesion is present in the distribution of a posterior inferior cerebellar artery, a vessel which normally arises directly from the vertebral (Fig. 32). It is clear from the above studies that the percentage of positive findings in patients with subarachnoid hæmorrhage increased progressively as the vascular investigation became more thorough and complete.

Bilateral carotid angiography is still desirable even where an aneurysm has been shown after the first carotid was injected. This is because about 5 per cent are found to have multiple aneurysms. In some patients more than two aneurysms have been demonstrated. When considering intracranial surgery or carotid ligation many neurosurgeons feel that it is important to have cross-compression

TABLE 8. PATHOLOGICAL FINDINGS AT VERTEBRAL ANGIOGRAPHY
FOR SUBARACHNOID HÆMORRHAGE

| | SPATZ AND BULL (60 cases) | SUTTON AND TRICKEY (77 cases) | | |
		GROUP II (UNILATERAL VERTEBRALS) (77 cases)	GROUP III (BILATERAL VERTEBRALS) (25 cases)	TOTAL VERTEBRALS 102 IN 77 PATIENTS
Aneurysms	8	16	6*	22*
Angiomas	8	10	2*	12*
Hæmatomas	0	2	0	2
Tumour	0	1	0	1
Negative	44	48	18	41

* One patient had both an aneurysm and an angioma.

angiographic studies in order to determine whether there is free flow across the anterior communicating artery. Such cross-compression studies are made by compressing one carotid artery whilst the other is injected with contrast. A freely patent anterior communicating artery will usually provide good contrast filling of the anterior and middle cerebral arteries on the contralateral side.

Techniques of Vertebral Angiography

Vertebral angiography can now be successfully and routinely achieved in all but exceptional cases by the judicious use of either needle or catheter technique, according to the patient and clinical problem.

In the past vertebral angiography has usually been performed by direct needle puncture from an anterior approach. Different workers tend to use different types of needles. Side-holed needles are

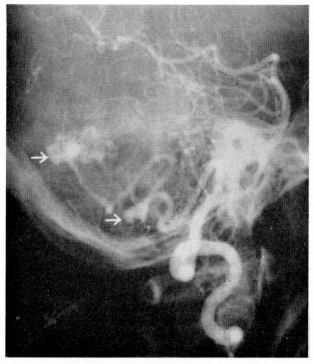

Figure 32. Aneurysm of the posterior inferior cerebellar artery.
(*Reproduced from Sutton and Trickey* (1962).)

advocated by some, but the author perfers to use an end-holed needle with a short sharp bevel. Most workers puncture the vessel in the mid or low cervical region with the needle fairly vertical; we prefer to puncture at a higher level with the needle at an angle of 45 degrees to the vertical.

The technique used is largely a matter of personal choice and experience. However, even in the most experienced hands, there is always a small percentage of failures and difficult punctures. This had led in recent years to an increasing interest in percutaneous catheter methods of vertebral angiography using the Seldinger technique. These methods have been modified over the years. The technique now favoured by the author is the right transaxillary approach and injection of the right vertebral artery. Sometimes a left transaxillary approach to the left vertebral is necessary. In younger patients the left vertebral can be approached from the groin by the simpler transfemoral catherization. The catheter is then passed straight up the aorta and into the left subclavian artery (Fig. 33).

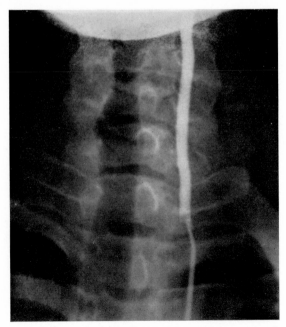

Figure 33.   Left vertebral arteriogram by percutaneous transfemoral catheterisation.

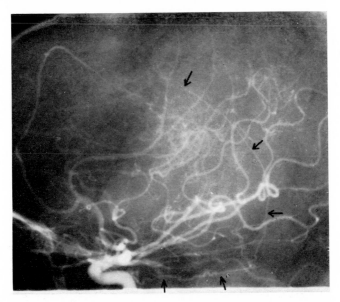

Figure 34. Tentorial branch of the internal carotid artery supplying a parasagittal tumour. These are usually meningiomas but in this case it was a glioma invading the falx.

However, catheter methods may fail to inject the left vertebral in cases where this vessel arises directly from the aortic arch, an anomaly occurring in 5 per cent of patients.

Tentorial Branches of the Internal Carotid Artery

Kramer and Newton (1965) reviewed previous descriptions of the tentorial branches of the internal carotid artery. These vessels are normally too small to be seen but lesions that involve the tentorium, particularly meningiomas, may enlarge them so that they are visualized at angiography.

In the lateral projection the tentorial artery arises from the proximal part of the carotid syphon lower down than the origin of the posterior communicating or anterior choroidal artery.

These tentorial arteries have mainly been demonstrated in cases of meningioma involving the tentorium though isolated examples have been reported with meningioma involving the falx. They have also been noted in some cases of angiomatous malformation, and in a few trigeminal neurinomas. There is an isolated report of the tentorial artery supplying a glioma, and we have personally encountered a similar case (Fig. 34). In these exceptional cases the glioma has presumably invaded the meninges and acquired a blood supply from them.

PNEUMOGRAPHY

Encephalography

In recent years there has been a greater tendency to use encephalography rather than ventriculography in the investigation of cerebral tumours, particularly those that lie in the posterior fossa.

Scandinavian workers showed some years ago that the sinister reputation of encephalography in this type of case was a result of

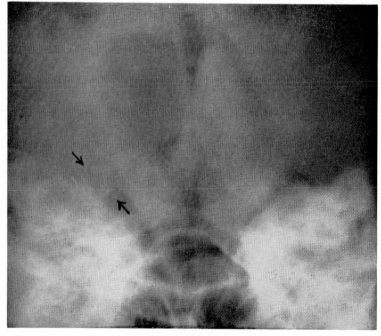

Figure 35.   Encephalogram showing a small acoustic tumour outlined by air in the cerebello-pontine angle.

faulty technique rather than an intrinsic defect of the method. Provided only small quantities of air are used, that the air is put in slowly and a corresponding amount of CSF is removed for each 4–5 ml injected there is little hazard attached to the procedure. Using as little as 10–15 ml of air a surprising amount of information can be obtained from the appearance of the air in the basal cisterns even if no air enters the ventricles (Fig. 35). If the aqueduct and 4th ventricle are adequately outlined further information can of course be obtained. Schechter *et al.* (1958) pointed out that even where the aqueduct and 4th ventricle have not been shown dilatation of the cisterna ambiens and of the cingulate gyrus cistern is usually strong evidence of the presence of a mass in the posterior fossa.

Pribram (1962) reviewed 15 confirmed posterior fossa tumours and observed that in addition to the signs noted by Schechter *et al.* (1958) other evidence of tumour may be shown. These include tonsillar herniation (outlined by a small amount of air in the cervical canal), flattening of the pontine cisterns, displacement of the

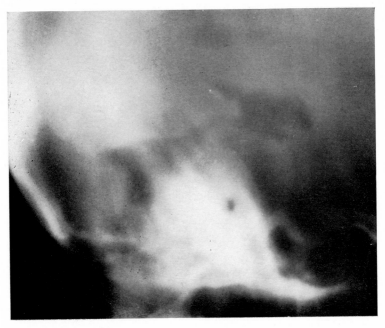

Figure 36. Autotomograms of the aqueduct and 4th ventricle.

quadrigeminal plate and outlining of the margin of an extracerebral tumour.

Tomography is being increasingly used with air studies and Di Chiro (1961a) has published a monograph on the subject. With the more sophisticated modern radiological apparatus tomography of the skull is possible without moving the patient's head. It is also possible to obtain "autotomograms" on simpler apparatus by having the patient slowly rotate his head during the X-ray exposure. With this technique excellent tomograms can be obtained of the midline structures of the brain, e.g. the anterior end of the 3rd ventricle, or the aqueduct and 4th ventricle (Fig. 36).

Diverticula of the Ventricles

Lorber and Grainger (1963) investigated a large number of children with hydrocephalus following tuberculous meningitis. They demonstrate that needling of the ventricles from the fontanelle was frequently followed by the development of diverticula from the ventricle extending upwards in the direction of the needle tract and giving rise to some odd ventricular appearances on later follow up. This work has also been confirmed in children with chronic hydrocephalus due to other causes.

Occult Hydrocephalus

Adams et al. (1965) described 3 cases which were clinically regarded as progressive presenile dementia. In all of these patients encephalography was performed and revealed what appeared to be a gross degree of ventricular dilatation. In all the cases the CSF pressure was within normal limits or doubtfully above what is regarded as the normal upper limit of 180 mm of water. The authors showed that all three patients were suffering from hydrocephalus despite the fact that the manometric pressures were not raised to the usual high levels.

The proof in these cases was provided by the fact that a shunting operation to relieve pressure or to reduce it to levels lower than the apparently normal levels produced a remarkable improvement in the symptoms and a restoration to almost normal mentality. One of the patients admittedly had a tumour in the third ventricle which was producing ventricular dilatation of the lateral ventricles. However, all clinical symptoms were relieved by the shunt operation and the patient was observed for at least two years following this operation with remarkable recovery to apparent normal mentality. The other two patients appeared to have some form of communicating hydrocephalus since the whole of the ventricular system was dilated. In these latter cases distinction must be made from irreversible cerebral atrophy where a similar encephalographic picture may be seen.

The authors make the point that with atrophy there is usually abundant air over the cortex. With the communicating low pressure hydrocephalus producing presenile dementia, air did not appear to pass over the cortex as in the atrophy cases.

This paper suggests that the accepted definition of what represents normal pressure in patients with presenile dementia due to atrophy should be re-evaluated and pressures of about or above 180 mm of water should be regarded as high. In these cases the air studies must be carefully evaluated before being accepted as showing "atrophy" and not hydrocephalus.

THE SPINE

Spinal Angiomas

Spinal angiomas were thought to be rather rare tumours but are now being diagnosed in increasing numbers. In the past diagnosis has been by myelography or by operative exposure. Angiomas may be extramedullary or intramedullary, or a combination of both. The hypertrophied vessels may be large or small and they may be arterial or venous. Diagnosis at myelography depends entirely on whether there are large vessels present which can be demonstrated as filling defects in the subarachnoid contrast material. Occasionally these are numerous and obvious. Sometimes, as with a large mainly intramedullary angioma, they may be few and difficult to demonstrate. In some cases it may be impossible to demonstrate the characteristic vascular shadows at myelography.

In recent years Houdart and Djindjian (1966) have shown that it is possible to demonstrate spinal angiomas directly. Since the angioma usually represents an arteriovenous communication without intermediate capillaries it is possible in many cases to show it by arteriography. The major vascular supply of the spinal cord is derived from the vertebral artery, and from the spinal branches of the lumbar arteries. The French workers have used thoracic and arch aortography to demonstrate angiomatous malformation of the spine. They use rather large doses of contrast medium and these are probably necessary to demonstrate angiomas fed by small arteries. They have shown that angiomas are often more extensive than the clinical features and myelographic studies would suggest.

Special arteriographic techniques may be helpful in demonstrating the smaller lesions and vessels. Biplane films or films taken in oblique projections are helpful. The vessels can also be better shown by the photographic technique of subtraction. This involves masking out the bony structures by a special photographic printing technique and leaving only the blood vessels standing out on the film. Since using angiography in the diagnosis of vascular disorders of the spinal cord Houdart and Djindjian have demonstrated 22 cases within three years. This proves conclusively that these lesions are much commoner than was previously thought.

Tonsillar Herniation

Tonsillar herniation in the frank Arnold-Chiari malformation has been well recognised for many years. Recently interest has been concentrated on minor degrees of cerebellar and tonsillar ectopia. It is now realised that many patients with symptoms suggesting a high cervical or medullary lesion are suffering from such minor lesions and that these can be associated with hydrocephalus. Diagnosis depends on careful myelography in the supine position with the object of outlining the lower borders of the tonsils and their relationship in the foramen magnum.

Discography

This technique permits radiographic visualization of the intervertebral discs utilizing direct injections of a water-soluble iodine containing contrast medium such as Hypaque. The intervertebral discs are enclosed by a dense fibrous ring, the annulus fibrosus. They contain a pulpy centre, the nucleus pulposus. Discography is performed either in the cervical or in the lumbar region in order to demonstrate prolapse of an intervertebral disc.

The needles are inserted into the discs under radiological control either by spot films or by fluoroscopy (preferably using an image intensifier). The cervical discs are approached from a lateral or anterolateral direction. The lumbar discs are approached from behind as for lumbar puncture. In either case the needle tip is inserted into the centre of the disc and this is confirmed by antero-posterior and lateral films or by screening. A small amount of a water soluble radiological opaque medium is then injected directly into the disc (Fig. 37). With a normal disc only about 0·5 ml of the contrast medium is required. A cervical disc appears as a single small pool of opaque medium. The lumbar disc however often has a biloculated appearance. Should there be a rupture of the annulus fibrosus then the contrast

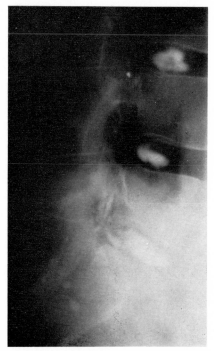

Figure 37. Discogram needles have been inserted into 3 lumbar discs showing a disc prolapse at L.5/S.1 and normal discs at L.2/3 and L.3/4.

medium is seen to escape posteriorly and up to 2 ml of contrast can be injected. This is confirmed by spot films. The contrast medium is slowly dispersed and has usually disappeared within half an hour.

There is a natural reluctance to puncture discs for fear of initiating a rupture, but protagonists of the method claim that such fears are groundless, and that the method is more accurate than myelography (Collis, 1962).

ULTRASONIC ENCEPHALOGRAPHY

The principles of echo-encephalography are similar to those developed during the war for localization of submarines (Asdic); they are also similar to the sound radar used by bats.

The use of sound for diagnosis in the basic form of percussion and auscultation is of course well known and long established. Ultrasonic diagnosis however employs sound waves whose frequency is far higher than can be registered by the human ear. Ultrasonic waves are produced from a transducer and travel through human tissue at a velocity of some 1,500 metres per second. When the wave reaches an object or surface with a different texture, or acoustic nature, a wave is reflected back from the surface of the object. These echoes are received back by the apparatus and changed into electric current. This can be amplified and shown on a cathode ray tube.

The use of echo-encephalography to measure the position of the

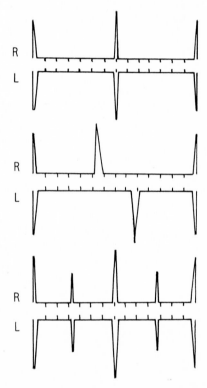

Figure 38. Normal echo-sound showing central midline structures.

Figure 39. Echo-sound showing marked shift of the midline structures to the right.

Figure 40. Diagram showing central mid line structures and echo from dilated ventricles in symmetrical hydrocephalus.

midline structures in the brain was first described by Leksell (1956). He showed that by passing a beam of pulsed ultra sound through the skull vault and recording the echoes produced he was able to detect the presence of displacement of the midline structures. This was later confirmed by many other workers and several clinical studies were published between 1958 and 1961.

Taylor *et al.* (1961) discussed the results of the ultrasonic technique in diagnosing the presence of a significant space-occupying lesion. The degree of accuracy of lateralization was 87 per cent in subsequently confirmed cases. Since then, work on these lines has continued in many centres with improvement in results.

Ford and Ambrose (1963) reviewed a series of one thousand consecutive echo-encephalographies, 867 of which were later confirmed by neuroradiological investigations. In these 867 confirmed cases 541 patients were considered to show no displacement of the midline structures and 326 patients were considered to show a displacement. 95·6 per cent of the patients thought to have no displacement were predicted correctly and 91 per cent of the patients thought to have a displacement were later shown to be correctly predicted. It is thus clear that in skilled hands the method can predict a shift of the midline structures with a very high degree of accuracy. This is obviously important in deciding the correct side for cerebral angiography to be performed in patients with doubtful or equivocal lateralizing signs.

Leksell (1956) also suggested that echo-encephalography might be useful in the diagnosis of hydrocephalus. This was because echoes could be obtained from the ventricular walls in cases where the ventricles were dilated. This suggestion was later confirmed by other workers.

Echo-encephalography has now become established as a valuable aid to the neurologist and neurosurgeon. It has proved to be a very satisfactory method of indicating the position of the diencephalic mid line and has several advantages in the screening of patients for further and more complex investigations by neuroradiology. The apparatus is very simple to use and causes no pain or discomfort to the patient.

The procedure can be performed on seriously ill or comatose patients and can also be performed at the bedside or elsewhere in the hospital. It is already of routine use.

1. In patients with head injury where intracerebral, subdural or extradural hæmatomas are suspected. A shift of the midline structures as shown by the echo-encephalogram will indicate the

presence of such a lesion and lateralize it prior to further investigation and treatment.

2. In patients with intracranial masses which are only vaguely or poorly localized by clinical methods the echo-encephalogram will again demonstrate whether or not there is a shift of the midline structures. In some cases this will indicate the correct side for carotid angiography and will save the patient an unnecessary investigation on the contralateral side. Thus many patients referred for "bilateral cerebral angiography" can be saved investigation of one side.

Figs, 38, 39 and 40 are simplified diagrams drawn from echo-encephalographic records to illustrate the points made in the above discussion. In each case the transducer or "probe" has been placed first against the right temple (upper record) and then against the left temple (lower record).

ISOTOPE ENCEPHALOGRAPHY

Isotope encephalography or "brain scanning," depends upon the injection of a radioactive isotope into the blood stream. The isotope is taken up by the cerebral tissue and there is a differential absorption in normal tissue and in neoplastic tissue. This fact enables tumours to be localized by an appropriate detector. The instrument is moved back and forth across the immobilized head producing a photographic scan or a print scan according to choice. The head is immobilized and two projections are usually taken at right angles to each other—a lateral and an anteroposterior as with conventional skull radiography. With most present day apparatus the procedure takes a considerable time and the head must be kept in a fixed position during the examination. Most patients tolerate this quite well but sedation is occasionally necessary in the more difficult patient. With the development of more sensitive apparatus much shorter scanning times will probably result and the so called "Gamma-Camera" seems to have now become a practical proposition.

Moore (1953) first described the localization of brain tumours by the use of gamma ray emitting substances.

He had previously shown that after intravenous injection sodium fluorescein was concentrated in brain tumours to a greater degree than in normal brain. He next tagged this compound with a radio-active element, [131]iodine, which emits gamma rays and these can easily be detected by means of a suitable detector pressed on the skull for external counting.

Since then considerable improvements and refinements have been made both in the apparatus used for detection of the radiation and in the substances injected intravenously to be taken up by the cerebral tumour. Di Chiro (1961b) published a monograph based on a study of a large number of cerebral tumours examined by isotope encephalography at the National Institute of Neurological Diseases and Blindness, Bethesda. About 400 patients had by this time been examined.

In the great majority of cases RISA (radio-active iodinated human serum albumen) was used as the gamma radiation source. Among the 400 cases there were 115 patients with verified intracranial lesions. In 95 cases the results of isotope encephalography were positive. In 20 cases false negatives were obtained. Thus a correct diagnosis was obtained in 84 per cent of the verified cases. These results were compared by Di Chiro with the results obtained by conventional radiological methods for the localization of intra cranial lesions and the results seemed very encouraging. Isotope encephalography was thus firmly established for the first time as an accepted and valuable method for neurological diagnosis. Since 1961 this important work has been confirmed from many other neurological centres.

In 1962 Blau and Bender introduced Neohydriol or Chlormedrin tagged with radio-active mercury (^{203}Hg) and this rapidly became popular as an agent for brain scanning. The isotope uptake at three hours is about double that provided by RISA at 24 hours. This gave it a considerable advantage for earlier and more effective detection and localization of intracranial lesions. Unfortunately, this substance is excreted by the kidneys and provides a relatively high radiation dose to them.

Sodee, Renner and Stefano (1965) suggested that ^{197}mercury might be more suitable for scanning of the brain and other organs. ^{197}Hg has a shorter half life and other advantages. Yamomoto, Feindel and Zanellie (1964) showed that it gave scans as satisfactory as those from Chlormedrin with ^{203}Hg and at the same time the radiation dose to the kidney was reduced to a negligible level. ^{197}Hg thus became, for a time, the radio isotope of choice for brain scanning. Later Technetium was proposed and used for this purpose and is proving to have considerable advantages even over ^{197}Hg (Harper *et al.*, 1965, McAfee *et al.*, 1964).

More recently Radioindium (^{113m}In) has been used (Stern *et al.*, (1967), Burrows *et al.*, (1968)). This isotope has a radio active half life of only 1.7 hours and the radiation dose to the patient is very much smaller than with other agents. This new product has given promising results which suggest that it may eventually become the radioisotope of choice for brain scanning.

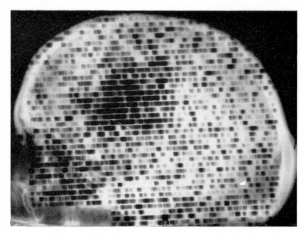

Figure 41*a*. Lateral brain scan showing heavy uptake of radio-active isotope (197Hs) in a posterior frontal tumour.

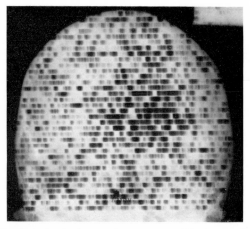

Figure 41*b*. Anterior brain scan in same case. The tumour is extending deeply and crosses the midline, indicating involvement of the corpus callosum (malignant glioma).

Interpretation of the brain scan requires familiarity with normal appearances. Thus certain areas always appear rather dark and show a higher uptake of isotope. These areas are located over the sinuses, mastoids, air cells and the suboccipital muscles in the lateral view. The sagittal sinus may also cause a ring or halo just over the skull vault in the lateral projection.

Istotope encephalography will usually detect masses larger than 2 cm. in diameter with a fair degree of ease. Smaller lesions however may be masked, particularly tumours with low grade malignancy. The more malignant tumours of course show more markedly positive scans (Figs. 41 and 42). The peripheral supratentorial tumours are the ones most readily detected. Deep seated tumours (for instance pituitary tumours) may not show on the brain scan. Posterior fossa tumours are also difficult to demonstrate because of the high uptake by the surrounding mastoid cells and suboccipital muscles. Occasionally however they may be quite well shown. Thus there are always a proportion of false negative results in patients with cerebral tumours investigated by this method.

On the other hand there may be false positive results with certain vascular lesions. Thus subdural hæmatomas may show quite a high uptake of isotopes. We have also seen false positive results in patients with unsuspected large aneurysms and with cerebral infarcts. Cerebral abscesses will also give positive scans, though the history will usually have suggested the diagnosis in these cases, and there is thus little likelihood of confusion with a tumour.

The more vascular tumours such as meningiomas and malignant gliomas show up much more readily on isotope examination than do non-vascular tumours. The situation of the tumour has often helped in suggesting a pathological diagnosis. Thus meningiomas may be parasagittal with their base up against the skull vault, or they may cross the falx, or be limited by it or the tentorium. Lesions crossing the midline in the region of the corpus callosum are usually gliomas involving this structure. This type of lesion is often very well shown by scanning.

Subdural hematomas may be suggested on the scan by their typical peripheral situation particularly when they prove to be bilateral.

Increased uptake with infarcts and vascular lesions tend to be well marked in the acute stage but may gradually return to normal on serial examination. The resolution of such lesions can be followed by scanning, as can the resolution of cerebral abscesses.

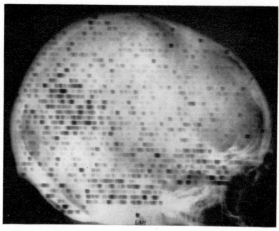

Figure 42. Lateral brain scan showing occipital pole tumour (glioma).

Scanning is particularly valuable in the diagnosis of secondary deposits since these may be multiple and small and they are often difficult to demonstrate by other methods.

RISA Encephalography

RISA (radio-active iodinated human serum albumen tagged with ^{131}I) can be injected into the subarachnoid space. In the normal patient the isotope diffuses up over the hemisphere of the brain and is absorbed within 48 hours. In patients with communicating or low pressure hydrocephalus the isotope passes into the ventricles and may be retained there for several days. Scanning of the head will demonstrate whether or not this is occuring and can be extremely useful in the diagnosis of this condition. Provided only a small dose of the isotope is used the radiation hazard seems to be well within tolerance limits (Bannister, Gilford, and Kocen, 1967).

References

ALPERS, B. J., BERRY, R. C., and PADDISON, R. M. (1964). *Arch. Neurol. Psychiat.*, **81**, 409.

ADAMS, R. D., FISHER, C. M., HAKIM, S., OJEMANN, R. G., and SWEET, W. H. (1965). *New Engl. J. Med.*, **273**, 117.

BANNISTER, R., GILFORD, E., and KOCEN, R. (1967). *Lancet*, **2**; 1014.

BLAU, M., and BENDER, M. A. (1962). *J. nuclear Med.*, **3**, 83.

BURROWS, E. H., KIMBER, P. M., and GODDARD, R. A. (1968). *Brit. M. J.* **2**: 29.

COLLIS, J. S. (1962). *Lumbar Discography*, Springfield, Ill., Charles C. Thomas.

DI CHIRO, G. (1961a). *An Atlas of Detailed Normal Pneumoencephalographic Anatomy.* Springfield, Ill., Charles C. Thomas.

DI CHIRO, G. (1961b). *Acta radiol. Stockh.* Supplement 201.

FORD, R., and AMBROSE, J. (1963). *Brain*, **86**, 189.

HAWKINS, T. D. (1966). *Clin. Radiol.*, **17**, 203.

HARPER, P. V., LATHROP, K. A., JIMINEX, F., FINK, R., and GOTTSCHALK, A. (1965). *Radiology*, **85**, 101.

HOUDART, R., and DJINDJIAN, R., (1966). *Proc. roy. Soc. Med.*, **59**, 789.

HUTCHINSON, E. C., YATES, P. O. (1956). *Brain*, **79**, 319.

KRAMER, R., and NEWTON, T. A. (1965). *Amer. J. Roentgenol.*, *Brain*, 826.

KUBIK C. S. and ADAMS, R. D. (1946) *Brain*, **69**, 73.

LEKSELL, L. (1956). *Acta chir. scand.*, **110**, 301.

LORBER, J., and GRAINGER, R. G. (1963). *Clin. Radiol.*, **14**, 98.

MCAFEE, J. G., FUEGER, C. F., STERN, H. S., WAGNER, H. N., and MAGITA, T. (1964). *J. nucl. Med.*, **5**, 811.

MOORE, G. E. (1953). *Diagnosis and Localization of Brain Tumours.* Springfield, Ill., Charles C. Thomas.

PRIBRAM, H. F. (1962). *J. Neurosurg.*, **19**, 269.

SCHECHTER, M. M., BULL, J. W. D., and CAREY, P. (1958). *Brit. J. Radiol.*, **31**, 317.

SODEE, D. B., RENNER, R. R., and STEFANO, B. D. (1965). *Radiology*, **84**, 873.

SPATZ, E. L., and BULL, J. W. D. (1957). *J. Neurosurg.*, **14**, 543.

STERN, H. S., GOODWIN, D., SCHEFFEL, V., WAGNER, H. N., and KRAMER, H. H. (1967). *Nucleonics*, **24**, 2: 62.

SUTTON, D., and TRICKEY, S. (1962). *Clin. Radiol.*, **13**, 297.

SUTTON, D., and DAVIES, E. R. (1966). *Clin. Radiol.*, **17**, 330.

TAYLOR, J. C., NEWELL J. A. and KARVOUNIS, P. (1961). *Lancet*, **1**, 1197.

WALSH, L. S. (1956). *Acta radiol. (Stockh.)*, **46**, 321.

WILLIAMS, D., and WILSON, G. (1962). *Brain*, **85**, 741.

WOLF, B. S., and YUN PENG HUANG (1964). *Amer. J. Roentgenol.*, **91**, 406.

YAMAMOTO, Y., FEINDEL, W., and ZANELLI, J. (1964). *Neurology (Minn.)*, **14**, 815.

INDEX